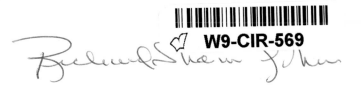

HEALING AFTER DARK

Pioneering Compassionate Medicine
at the
Boston Evening Clinic

A Memoir by

Morris A. Cohen, M.D.

**Recollections, Introduction, Epilogue, Index,
and Editing by Richard Shain Cohen**

Additional Editing by Helen Compton

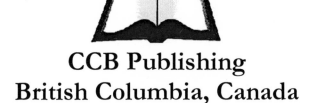

CCB Publishing
British Columbia, Canada

Healing After Dark:
Pioneering Compassionate Medicine at the Boston Evening Clinic

Copyright ©2011 by Richard Shain Cohen
ISBN-13   978-1-926918-44-0
First Edition

Library and Archives Canada Cataloguing in Publication
Cohen, Morris A. (Morris Aaron), 1893-1974
Healing after dark : pioneering compassionate medicine at the Boston Evening Clinic : a
memoir / by Morris A. Cohen ; recollections, introduction, epilogue, index and editing by
Richard Shain Cohen ; additional editing by Helen Compton.
Includes Index.
ISBN 978-1-926918-43-3 (bound).--ISBN 978-1-926918-44-0 (pbk.)
Also available in electronic format.
1. Boston Evening Clinic--History.
2. Clinics--Massachusetts-- Boston--History.
3. Cohen, Morris A. (Morris Aaron), 1893-1974.
4. Physicians--Massachusetts--Boston--Biography.
5. Poor--Medical care--Massachusetts--Boston--History.
I. Cohen, Richard Shain II. Title.
RA982.B72B67 2011   362.1'20974461   C2011-902390-3

United States Copyright Office Registration # TXu 889-873

Richard Shain Cohen may be contacted through: **www.richardshaincohen.com**

Publisher: CCB Publishing
             British Columbia, Canada
             www.ccbpublishing.com

DEDICATION

To Morris A. Cohen's grandsons: Myles J. Cohen, M.D.; Martin I. Cohen, M.D.; and Mylan C. Cohen, M.D., M.P.H. Each of them would make their grandfather proud of their dedication to their patients and for their accomplishments in their chosen fields of medicine.

Also, to all those doctors, and staff, who aided my father in making the Boston Evening Clinic the outstanding institution it was under his direction.

And may Morris' great-grandchildren learn the lessons in life taught by him: compassion, humility, kindness, and service for the betterment of society.

– Richard S. Cohen

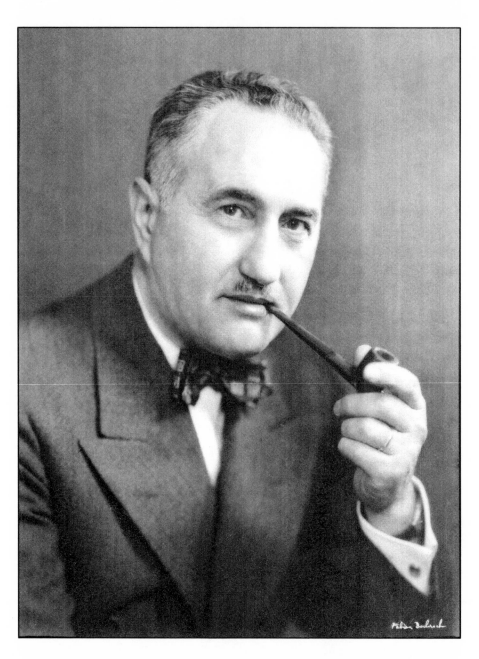

Portrait: Morris A. Cohen, M.D.

CONTENTS

ACKNOWLEDGEMENTS

Thanks go to Mylan C. Cohen, M.D., M.P.H. who a number of years ago helped with editing the beginning of the book.

I acknowledge with thanks the following books from which there are brief borrowed passages:

Means, Dr. J. Howard. *Doctors People And Government.*

Folsom, Marion. *Health Care Is A Community Affair.*

Harrington, Michael. *The Other America* and *USA Today.*

Others who have my gratitude include the following:

Publications for permission to use quotes from their papers: *The Boston Globe, The Boston Herald, The New York Times,* and *The Jewish Advocate. The Boston Sunday Advertiser* provided a short quote.

I am grateful to Jack Kennealy for providing a number of photographs in the book, including the cover photo of Morris A. Cohen's medical bag, pipe, and ash tray, the latter as they appeared on his office desk.

And I must acknowledge my indebtedness to Helen Compton who designed the cover and edited the book so diligently and intelligently. Helen died in 2010 after a terrible auto accident.

– Richard S. Cohen

INTRODUCTION

It took years of maturing to realize that my father, Morris A. Cohen, M.D., was, in a sense, a man who had to do unpleasant work because others wouldn't such as Atticus Finch out of the pages of Harper Lee's magnificent novel, *To Kill A Mockingbird*. My father's story is one that I learned while growing up, watching the Boston Evening Clinic grow with me, listening to stories told by my father and the family, reading newspapers, listening to criticism of him that embarrassed me — but realizing that those critics were wrong, and that my father was a man of whom to be proud, for he followed his instinct for what was right and humane in this life. The lessons he tried to teach me included the importance of humility, lack of pretension, and appreciation of those who suffer, financially and for other reasons. Early on he took me to the slums of Boston where he visited patients — white, black, Asian — who lived in dwellings with falling plaster. Although I grew up in comfort, the images of the people in the Clinic and in those tenements engraved themselves into me and will never leave. My recognition of my father's worth came with difficulty, for his mission was carried out at some cost to our family life. I was young enough when the struggle played out that my admiration and loyalties were severely tested. Yet, when old enough to know who my father was and what he was, I knew a pride in him that will also never be lost.

The story is an amazing one, for neighborhood clinics and help for the poor that you see today were unknown and unavailable when Morris Cohen started his medical practice. With the founding of the Boston Evening Clinic, my father pioneered the concept of compassionate medicine for the lower-income person, probably for the first time in the nation, according to many articles that appeared in the newspapers of the time. And frankly, he had to fight like hell to do it. Eventually he won the labor unions and finally the Medical Society; then money started to come in — but never enough. He never gave up. As time passed and people realized what he was doing, his Clinic became well known. John F. Kennedy sat on an advisory board before becoming President and was influenced by the Clinic's work. Edward Kennedy supported the Clinic, of course, and it is to my father's honor in a small way that last year saw the Health Care Reform Bill for which Senator Ted fought so hard and so long. And others came also — Tom Dooley had a partner who came. The Lord Mayor of Dublin appeared. When Johnson was President, he invited Morris to the White House Conference on Health. And so on.

The following article was printed in *The Boston Herald* on June 27, 1964:

---

37 Years of Aid to Ailing: Million Treated By Evening Clinic

The Boston Evening Clinic established in 1927 to treat the working man and his family when they can spare the time to come, is reaching its 1,000,000 patient mark.

When the clinic was established 37 years ago by Dr. Morris A. Cohen, the still active medical director, some 1,000 patients were helped in the first 12 months.

Now this unique medical service station — world famous for "healing after dark" — treats more than 20,000 persons each year. The total number of "admissions" is well over the 900,000 mark.

More than 50 doctors serve in 20 different departments providing medical care for almost all ailments. Some of the special departments include cancer detection, heart disease, arthritis, dental, allergies and psychiatric care.

Because it makes available a wide range of medical services normally obtainable only during the daytime, thousands of persons requiring attention are able to receive it without loss of time from work, without loss of pay, without the added financial burden of private medical care and without adding to the problem of absenteeism in industry.

For this reason, the clinic, perhaps the most complete evening medical service in the country, is supported by both business and labor. It offers treatment to those who don't want charity and can't afford the working time to visit other medical facilities. It has saved employers millions of valuable manpower hours by treating employees in the evening . . .

As the clinic approaches their million mark, its purpose as originally expressed by Dr. Cohen remains the same: "To create a haven for the ailing and depressed, where all alike find an atmosphere in which human dignity and self-respect are preserved."

Another article which appeared in the same paper states:

In this era of the Organization Man to whom the single courageous act for an untested idea is not only outlandish but outmoded, it is exciting to see and give recognition to that rare individualist who is willing to go it alone for something he believes in. Such an individual is Dr. Morris A. Cohen: founder, medical director and guiding spirit of the Boston Evening Clinic . . .

The idea of after dark medical centers is now finding wide acceptance. But for three and one half decades, Dr. Cohen, with obstinacy and perseverance, pioneered this vital concept.

Today the Boston Evening Clinic is among the foremost full-time evening clinics in the United States, offering a complete range of medical and surgical care, five evenings a week, at less than cost fees and often at no cost at all, for hundreds of thousands of working people and their families in Greater Boston.

If such efforts were possible then — for example, the Clinic later worked in conjunction with the Boston University School of Medicine and the then Boston City Hospital — one must ask how it is possible today that all people are not treated regardless of cost. Again, our elected officials, the insurance companies, many national politicians, and some in the medical establishment will not allow it. Look back to the Clinton years and the contemptible *Harry and Louise* ads. In fact, one year Dr. Cohen approached The Massachusetts General Hospital (which was in the news for its covert arrangement with a very prominent insurance company of the area) for a working relationship, but the hospital decided against an affiliation with the Clinic. In the late 1990s, however, it purchased the Clinic, because the City of Boston forced hospitals to provide such care in the community. There will be more of this story in the pages that follow.

There have been and continue to be efforts at establishing evening centers in Boston. There is Women of Means, started by Dr. Roseanna Means, for homeless and indigent women, and children. In 2010 a group of retired physicians gathered to repeat what my father started in 1927. One of Boston's outstanding Rabbis also called on hospitals to work toward community health. I am willing to suggest that neither the group of caring physicians nor the Rabbi had any idea of the history that took place before their efforts. There are now two such clinics in Portland, Maine. It is astounding that there are people calling for what was already in existence over eighty years ago through the will of one man who realized the purpose of his profession. The following are in Dr. Cohen's own words, written between 1966-1967:

"*Although I have repeatedly praised organized medicine and its representatives for their great contribution to medical science, I do believe my story must be completely objective and not be distorted by glossing over what is not praiseworthy [in the profession]. . . . I am . . . writing [also] in the hope of inspiring others to the service of humankind.*"

Morris Cohen never intended to be an author, never desired to write this story. But in 1966 or 1967, among others, Clement Stone, a wealthy man who gave money to the Clinic, persuaded him that it ought to be told.

Here, then, follows in Dr. Morris A. Cohen's words the almost unbelievable story of the Boston Evening Clinic and of a man with the fortitude and courage to withstand the withering attacks of the Boston medical establishment, including even the Massachusetts Medical Society. It is a matter of disgrace — and honor — that the medical field finally realized what Dr. Cohen had the foresight to accomplish from 1927 until his death in 1974. Occasionally my own memories and comments will interject, with the intent not to distract from his story but to fill it in with the scenes and clarifications he left out in order to shine the light where he felt it ought rightfully to be, on the Clinic and the American citizens whose lives and health it saved.

— Richard S. Cohen

CHAPTER ONE: BEGINNINGS

This memoir is not primarily the story of my life but rather a narrative of commitment made during my youth to a mission. Undoubtedly, certain episodes of my childhood gave rise to my eventual new ideal in medical care. I founded the Boston Evening Clinic and Hospital for the indigent and for workers who were unable to seek care during the day because time off for health reasons could cost them wages, and for those who did not and still do not have sufficient funds for more expensive or specialized care. The medical establishment, banks, and other organizations, as you will read, fought the clinic but could not stop me or its work — which grew until on December 13, 1964, *The New York Times* included an article commemorating the millionth admittance. A short quote indicates the significance of the struggle: *"A Boston physician [Morris A. Cohen] anticipated President Johnson's declaration of war on poverty and disease, 37 years ago."*

Therefore, heedful that this story is that of the Boston Evening Clinic and Hospital, that story is ill told unless I particularize the moments in my life that compelled me to commit myself to this task.

At the outset, I wish to make it clear that these are not reminiscences written in tranquil retirement years. Still engaged full time in all of my work as Medical Director of the Boston Evening Clinic now in 1967, at the age of 74, my life does not normally allow me time for looking backward. I have repeatedly declined the urging of friends to document publicly the adversities that were attendant upon the establishment of this Institution because of its extraordinary growth. Only now have I at last been persuaded by family and some clinic benefactors to tell the story.

One of the themes — a belief to which my life attests — is

that we must reaffirm the value of truth and altruism and their rewards. We must reawaken the incentive and courage to give of ourselves, for it is only in giving that we truly receive what is most worthwhile. This record I set down has relevance and inspiration for anyone seeking to achieve today. My story is timely, and it convincingly shows that environment, experience, responsibility, discipline, and conduct are determinants in shaping one's character and success.

While I have repeatedly praised organized medicine and its representatives for their outstanding contributions to medical science, I do believe my story must be completely objective and not be distorted by glossing over what is not praiseworthy. It is my intention not to hide the activities carried out to undermine the establishment of the Clinic but to present the obstacles in their fullness for an absolutely realistic picture of events.

One of my purposes is to create public awareness and confidence in the public's ability to attain enhancement in medical service, as well as to demand the cooperation of fellow citizens in obtaining the improvements in delivery whenever they are not provided by existing agencies. This extends to Congress and the presidency and to established institutions, as well as to the industries that would prevent full medical care because of desire for more and more profit. It is obstacles such as the latter two that I faced but through which I endured. If a single individual can succeed, what may an entire population accomplish? As an example, I believe I must boldly express a critical judgment of the action of organized medicine which nearly eliminated, for example, our pioneer establishment of the Boston Evening Clinic's Cancer Detection Center.

It is incredible that adequate medical care should be shunted aside because of ideology, greed, or indifference.

President Johnson had said, "Our national resources for health have grown, but our national aspirations have grown faster. Today we expect what yesterday we could not envision: adequate care for every citizen." Congress, because of the President, passed a controversial act. While some of us in medicine looked favorably upon this, others in our field opposed the establishment of Medicare, which assured adequate health care at least for one large deserving segment of Americans — those over 65. Some of us see this as an improvement too long postponed, since America's health care standard falls below that already developed by other western countries.

So, what events brought me to this point of revelation and action? Well it is with joyous memories that I look back to my early life, despite my birth under conditions of persecution and oppression in Romania. I was born in the town of Podu-Iloi in 1893, in a two-room mud-wall shack. A big iron kettle was set in the dirt floor. Meals were cooked in that one pot, the family eating while seated on the floor around the pot.

Families there lived within a compound, with dwellings arranged in a semi-circle for better protection. In the center were two main houses for the elders. As the elders passed on, the next in age moved up to these houses. In winter, the children kept warm by sleeping on a squared-off portion of the floor near the stove-warmed wall.

Oh, the weddings and the feasts we had! Those were wonderful times, when a canvas was thrown across both main houses and when the great area of the compound was filled with tables for feasts, and gypsies came and played music. I well remember one of the weddings in the winter, when the only way you could get out of the house was by digging a tunnel through the high mounds of snow to get into the street, and the men with a four-horse drawn sleigh went out to gather guests for the wedding. Afterwards came the gypsy music, and there was dancing all night in the snow-filled streets. So you may see that there *were* joys of youth to remember.

Beyond the music, every Monday at dawn, my father — with a carbine across his shoulder, pistol in his boot, and knife in his belt — set out to go to distant farms to buy grain, which would be delivered by the farmers on Sunday-market days and then stored in grain barns within the family compound. He was heavily armed for possible encounters with bandits who would not hesitate to rob and murder an unarmed man.

Yes, we had bad men, and we had teenage difficulties too, but they were exciting times for the young. The town was divided by a river, which gave it its name: *Podu* — bridge of the river, and *Iloi* — the river's name. The boys' gang organized from above the river always met on the bridge to fight the gang from below the river. We rode into the fight like the old Romans, using reins and harnessed to a boy "horse" in front of us. The "horse" made certain we would not retreat. We met there on the bridge with pikes and sticks and stones until one group or the other retired. Far be it for me to say one or the other was ever "vanquished." And I must say also that those from the lower section of the city — our side — were the toughest gang.

These were also my grammar school years when every four months the teacher, a reserve army officer, was rushed to the Bulgarian border because of frequent military clashes there. But these youthful excitements ended with completion of grammar school at age ten when, for the first time, I was called upon by necessity to become a supporting member of the family. I did this both willingly and confidently. I went to work as a salesman in a dry goods store in the big city of Jassy. I have never forgotten watching — from the sidewalk of the big city — the Queen's cavalry marching out from the city of Jassy to the town of Podu-Iloi, where my parents and family still lived, to quell riots and initiate pogroms against us Jews. I was told that the Jewish male population built a stockade fort to defend itself while waiting until the cavalry came. Perhaps I romanticize, but it is no wonder to me that with this background, the picture of my father with a bandolier makes me think of bandits or of the cavalry riding to the rescue in John Ford movies. Is it any wonder I love the movies of the Old West, of the Native Americans, the cowboys, the pioneers? With a boy's pride I remember my father, dressed in Romanian peasant clothing, riding with fast horses and carriage through the little villages to carry the family to town for safety.

As the pogroms continued, the government ordered all Jewish families to move out of their small communities and villages. That meant we had to leave home, to seek salvation and renewal in any country that would accept us into its society as free people. At that time, we knew that to be true of only Canada and the United States of America. Romania would become a foreign country to us, later even more foreign under Communism.

It is with horror that I contemplate what might have happened to my father and his family if they had NOT emigrated. In the area of Jassy, the city where my father worked as a pre-teen, the pogroms he described continued to flare up and ended in 1941 as a brutal slaughter of what remained of the 50,000 Jews residing there, which amounted to fifty percent of the population.

— Richard S. Cohen

My memories of leaving home and all possessions except what we could carry are the vivid ones of an alert twelve year old. Leaving Romania behind forever, we journeyed by train to Vienna, Berlin, and finally took steerage passage in, by today's standards, a small boat, the *Parisienne* out of Southampton. The giant waves terrified me, reaching so far above the boat. The appalling conditions of steerage passage were equally shocking: everyone lived and slept en masse on the floor. As for meals, we ate what we had brought with us.

Our family group landed in Montreal: six children, an aunt and her two children, and a grandmother, who lived long enough to see me a year into the practice of medicine, and who was eased and grateful for her grandson's ministrations in her last illness. Canada had offered to immigrants free land for farming — but my father, finding that it was all rocky soil, decided after two weeks to move on. I guess we did not quite measure up to the pioneers who went westward.

So, by invitation of my father's sister in Boston, we came to that city on a day in September, 1907, where she welcomed us to her five room apartment on Leverett Street. Here we were settled, housed, fed, and began a new life in a new country.

My father immediately had to find a way to support his growing family. My mother was seven months pregnant. An uncle, his brother-in-law, helped my father buy a horse and team to peddle vegetables. We rented an unheated basement apartment on Auburn Street, in the West End of Boston. From the selling of vegetables, after paying for food and keep of horse and team, my father brought home about five dollars a week net. My grandmother, the toughest of the gang, did all the cooking and took care of all the children. I was the oldest. I spoke some English but the others didn't.

The first item on the agenda: It was mandatory in the United

States to go to school. Because of my previous grade school education in Romania, including the study of German, and with my broken English, the administration placed me in the first grade one morning, the third that afternoon, and by the next year in the fifth.

I not only had to attend school but also had to become a contributor to help support the family. In those days, at my age, it meant one thing — selling newspapers. Therefore, before school, during lunch hour, after school, and, of course all Saturday night, I sold papers.

To sell papers successfully and to make a large enough profit to benefit the family meant owning a corner. The only key to owning one was street toughness. Like gangsters of old, the idea was to take over — to knock out the fellow who already had the corner. I well remember the beatings I took every morning until I learned how to defend myself. (The fighting on the bridge in Romania hadn't prepared me for what I now faced.) I had to fight to defend my own corner and so I did. The corner that was to become mine was Brattle Street, in Scollay Square at the subway station where I would sell from sunrise until school time. That corner belonged to another boy who used it during school hours. If you owned the corner and allowed another boy to sell, the boy owner stood beside him and kicked him in the shins to make him keep screaming "Extra! Extra! Extra! *Herald, Globe, Record, Traveler,* and *American!*" So we sold the papers by screaming "Extra." The big "Extras" in those days were highway robbers. I, not quite knowing what the words meant, yelled, "High May Robbery!"

Also at about this time, we joined what I believe was the first newsboy strike, which was against the *Morning Journal*. We did not yell that paper's name. We had to join the strike, or else. I don't remember nor do I believe I ever knew what the strike was about, primarily because I did not know English well enough. I *did* realize that if I sold the *Journal,* I would be battered.

Years later I reminisced with the publisher of *The Boston Globe* about these early times of selling. We talked of how we would sell the first edition of *The Globe* from about two a.m. to six a. m., going after the all-night workers. Then, at 6 a.m., when the subway opened, we would wait for the morning riders and sell until almost school time, when we would eat breakfast in Pie Alley at Gridley's. There for ten cents you could have beans, pie, coffee, cereal, and toast or rolls — an elaborate meal at a price well within our means.

Winters were the worst. There was no daily snow removal. It piled quite high on the streets and sidewalks. On those freezing mornings, we had to hold out the papers in our numbed hands to display the headlines. Gloves were an impossible luxury.

Families were also an expense, but that mattered little, especially if they were close and depended upon one another. In the early part of the century, families had a way of enlarging, regardless of any inability to provide for them. Another baby was on the way. That would make eight children, a grand-mother, and an aunt. The cellar apartment just wasn't large enough — we had to move. Because my father had not earned much more in his new trade, we moved to a dark alley of Cushman Avenue, between Chambers and Leverett Streets of the West End. The only light was a gas jet.

And we required more money to support all of us. That was the tragedy of my young life, for the only solution was for me to leave the fifth grade and get full time work. I found a job in a little store on Brattle Street so I could continue selling papers in the morning and on Saturday nights. I worked at that store for only five days. On the fifth day, the owner handed me a broom to sweep the sidewalk. For the first time, I became aware of my ambition; sweeping sidewalks would not give me the future I envisioned. Instead, my situation became a challenge; challenge breeds incentive; incentive, if strong enough, always finds a way. I took that broom and started for the sidewalk but instead of sweeping, I gently but determinedly placed it against the wall of the store and walked home. I never returned for my pay, determined instead that I must go to school.

The question now was how to serve my newfound pride and ambition under what were to me impossible circumstances — the sacrifice of half my earnings. I solved the problem by deciding to become an employer and began a new life of individual enterprise. Rather than fighting, I bought out the newspaper corner from the boy who owned it during the day and also hired another to sell on the corner after I left in the morning for school. I became a capitalist. Yes, I returned to the fifth grade and then found myself in the seventh in the middle of the school year. I was not only succeeding in school, but I also was a leading contributor to the family's economic welfare. Moreover, I could speak English rather well by now, but more importantly, I had already laid the first stones toward the fulfillment of my dream to build my own way of life.

I cannot continue without memorializing that famous newspaper corner, my personal foundation, by mentioning that there, fifty feet away from me at the corner of Cornhill and Court Streets, two other boys cried, "Extra!" — Alexander Brin and his younger brother, Joseph. Alexander became the publisher of *The Jewish Advocate* and Joseph, Professor of Semantics at Boston University. Our close friendship has lasted, though now Joseph has passed away.

All too often people have heard, "My children will have a better life than I did." So it was with many of my generation who adhered to these teachings and beliefs. It is safe to say that many of the professionals who are or were of my generation came from humble beginnings.

That newspaper corner and other early experiences from my youthful life had to have impelled me toward, and nurtured in me, individual enterprise. I see free enterprise as the fountainhead of initiative, the foundation of a productive America. Often I have wondered about and answered this question, *"Did we bring rugged individualism with us, or did we acquire it here in a country in which we found freedom, opportunity, and inspiration to become citizens who would enrich the country by cherishing and perpetuating its way of life?"*

My answer is that opportunity is not born full grown. It arrives at one's door to become a guest of the one who answers. With opportunity is challenge. These guests may cause doubt or fear, but both these unsettling emotions must be put aside, shed like the winter boots guests remove when coming indoors. One must be willing to pay the price necessary for achievement.

However, it would also be preferable if all people recognized — as I do — that opportunity which brings a better life also requires a concern for others. We owe dedication to the work we offer, but greater dedication of our talent should be devoted to helping others as we perform the work we love. Thus, freedom and the ability to provide for oneself must also include joint community effort and kinship with one's neighbors — a real concern for one's companion human beings. It is this that our immigrant parents taught us, as well as the need for knowledge. We were taught the necessity of completing our education and of becoming trained to be professional servants of the community. Our parents, lacking the fortunes to start us in large business ventures, had the conviction that a profession — for example that of physician, architect, lawyer — meant a valuable life for, as I have said, both personal gain and for community benefit.

By choosing those professions we were also repaying the United States for its gift of citizenship to us who came from so many different lands. This motivation was aptly affirmed recently by Chief Justice Elijah Adlow in a speech before the West End Old Timers at the Somerset Hotel. He stated: "Whether they came from Ireland, Eastern Europe, or Italy, they came with a determination to prove themselves worthy of America." I distinctly recall having this feeling as a youth. What one must recognize is that the United States placed the opportunities and the professions within our reach. It was never primarily for fame and fortune. The education we sought and professions we chose were for the purpose of making us respectable members of American society, thereby enabling us to enrich and improve the greater community.

Segregation? Discrimination? We had experienced that in other lands. We also experienced it here. There were troubles, and unfortunately there was violence; however, rebellion and more violence would not correct these injustices. No. Most of us knew that faith in ourselves and hard work were the answers, the keys to advancement.

Because of such feelings, I look back at those who were in our Boston West End neighborhood and see judges of Superior and Supreme Courts. An example is Judge Higgins who played craps with me at the corner of Green and Chardon Streets in front of the Hendrix Club. There are so many others who have become well-known physicians, surgeons, and nationally and internationally prominent attorneys. I learned therefore, early on, that there is a dynamic force generated by human dignity that thereafter invests successful efforts with a spirituality. Accordingly, my choice of profession would be one of service, through which I could give. As far as I am concerned, the profession at the top of the list is that of physician. Who can serve people better than a healer?

I have described my economic arrangements during youth, and now I had to ask, because I had made a choice of schooling, *"Is it going to be hard, perhaps an impossible undertaking?"* I decided cost was not a limiting factor, that it could not be. Besides, my family was now experiencing some financial relief. I had completed grammar school and was now in high school; my aunt had married and moved away; my father earned more, six or seven dollars a week. Two of my brothers were now selling newspapers.

Yet, people have a way of making things harder for themselves. In my second year at English High School (a huge Victorian structure on Warren Street for male students only) I had a steady girlfriend, Anna Shain, who was to become my first wife and mother of our five children. In those days one did not go with a girl unless it was on a steady basis, according to parental dictate. I was just a little over eighteen.

Well, at that time, to take a girl for a ride, you took a horse and carriage. My father and uncle each had a horse and wagon because they were both in the business of peddling. They kept these at Charles Street stables. One Sunday I hired a carriage and chose my uncle's horse, a more handsome one than my father's. I did not ask permission, just took the horse. In the evening, Anna and I were returning and riding on Chambers Street when my uncle saw me with his horse pulling the carriage. All day he had been wildly running about looking for the horse. Anna had just stepped from the carriage, and as I turned from helping her down, I felt a slap on my face. My uncle was on the carriage, repeatedly hitting me. Of course, you did not strike your elders in defense. He did not ask why I took the horse. I just accepted that I was going to pay his price — a good beating. Just about then, a policeman came along, grabbed my uncle to stop the beating, and asked what I had done. Without hesitation, my uncle screamed, "He stole my horse!" The officer asked if the horse was his. I told him it was. So I had my second ride that day: I was taken off the carriage and to the Joy Street Police Station, while my uncle took his horse and the carriage back to the stable. The officer lodged me in the basement of the station, a dark and filthy place where I sat wretchedly, believing I would forever be branded a horse thief. Aren't I lucky this hadn't happened out west? I could very well have been dangling from a tree. That would have been frontier days in Boston.

In our neighborhood every incident, every action was, by instinct almost, a *community* action. Thus, within half an hour after I was left in the cell, *all* the friends, *all* the neighbors were at the police station pleading with my uncle to realize what he was charging me with. My uncle felt nothing more strongly than fear for himself, for he would have to find a good reason for beating me and for being the cause of my jailing. In about three hours, my family bailed me out. My uncle had disappeared. All night my father stormed up and down the streets looking for his brother. He did not find the frightened man. Next morning, everything was explained to the judge. The horse thief label was at least legally removed, but the shame remained with me for some time.

On the home front, with steady financial progress, the family was able to rent a five room flat in Brighton Court that was not quite so dark as Cushman Avenue. This apartment had a gas jet in each room, but it was still necessary for some children to sleep on the floor. The time had also come for me to begin making definite plans for my schooling, and Anna and I were developing plans for marriage. With these advancing ambitions, there was a need for greater earnings. To do what I wanted, I bought the newsstand in the Crawford House and also began to sell papers all night at Adams Square. That was a combined enterprise!

The family now moved to Lowell, Massachusetts and started its new business, a small bakery. Entering my third year of high school, I could not join my family, so I went to live with the Levine family — of whom Joseph Levine, later to become famous in the movie industry, was one of three sons and two daughters. We still slept on the floor, and there were no baths. Therefore on Sunday mornings family groups would go to the North End public bathhouse where for one cent we could take showers. Imagine my sensations on Sunday mornings, after selling papers all night, when I was awakened by the clangor of pots and pans that were beaten to awaken everyone for the weekly trip to the bathhouse.

Because of my plans for further education and marriage, I had to earn more. Thus, the way of capitalism and free enterprise. I bought a little tobacco store on Friend Street near North Station. A still further venture was a partnership with Sam Grover, who later became a dentist and who is still in practice. We hired a horse and team to sell produce in Faneuil Hall Market. For this work, we had to draw police lots for a place in line. What should we sell? We decided upon discarded barrels of candies, like the seconds some stores now sell, that came from stores such as the five and dimes once so prevalent. Loading the teams with barrels, we sold the candy by the pound, making a net profit of ten dollars each. That was a large sum to add to my other earnings. An indisputable successful financier at nineteen years old, I proposed. The Shains agreed to the marriage, which took place on January 13, 1913. Then, to ensure the continuation of my studies, we moved in with

Anna's parents on Chambers Street. With but small contributions for rent and food, it was possible to continue my education.

CHAPTER TWO: A MEDICAL MAN

Nothing interfered with my determination to study medicine. There being no classification of medical schools in those days, I would choose a smaller medical college which charged less and that would also allow me time to work the necessary hours to earn tuition. It was beginning to look as though the task was monumental. And dilemmas multiplied: we were to have our first child. It appeared there were terrible decisions to be made. I lacked sufficient savings for medical school but would have to give up some of my working hours and earnings. There was an additional pressure: consideration of whether or not to leave school. I would not be interrupting my desire to study as much as abandoning a dream. I could not do this. I chose to finish high school by taking night classes. On being graduated, I took the examination at the medical school, passed, and was admitted.

On September 7, 1913, our first son, Manley, was born. He would later graduate from Harvard and become a physician; after the war he continued with his training in thoracic surgery and practiced in El Paso, Texas. Yet, he would unfortunately die a young man. How does one explain the death of a child or comfort oneself? Time does not heal as well as many believe, but there are so many proud and happy memories — on June 6, 1967, I was present to see Manley's son Myles receive his medical degree from Columbia School of Medicine.

How did I hope to do so much in days containing too few hours? Determination. Once in medical school, my time and labor had to be carefully apportioned among study, work, and family. I arranged for the first and second years. By the third year, though, I would not only attend classes but would spend mornings in clinical work at Boston City Hospital. It was necessary to give up personally selling papers while keeping the Crawford House News and Tobacco stand, as well as the little tobacco store. I also started selling the *Standard Dictionary of Facts* house-to-house in what spare time there was. Summer was also a time to earn still more for all the necessary expenses.

Among those who helped in my businesses was Samuel Kamberg, who became a noted radiologist, and my brother Sol — who was to become a Hollywood agent for stars such as George Jessel and Zazu Pitts — and who tragically died at a young age of a brain tumor. Despite the advancing knowledge we had in the late 1920s, there was nothing that could yet be done to help or to save him.

Some medical students at that time found summer work at a machine factory in South Ashburnham. I did not think that job would bring enough for the summer, so I acquired work as a motorman on an open streetcar that ran from Fall River, Massachusetts to Providence, Rhode Island. The line was a single track which ran alongside the road in what you might call the walk sections of towns and fields. As a spare motorman at twenty-five cents an hour and wanting more, I waited around the car barn that was on a hill in Fall River hoping to get additional hours. While in Fall River, I got word from the bunch in South Ashburnham that they had gotten a large barn on a hill outside town which they used for sleeping quarters. It belonged to the owner of the Waldorf Restaurant chain. According to my friends they could exist on two dollars a week and still have enough to save. That settled it for me — the next day I was on my way to South Ashburnham where a job was waiting for me.

How did we manage on two dollars a week? My father had moved back from Lowell and now owned a grocery store in Cambridge. Every week he sent us a barrel of bread, vegetables, and milk in ten-quart cans. By haying on weekends for the local farms, we received eggs and other staples. So we were able to save money. And we students became machinists overnight: the United States was now engaged in World War I, so every man — experienced or not — could find work that aided the war effort, much like later in World War II when the women went to work in such numbers. The only machines we couldn't use were the automatic ones, because of our inexperience. What we were allowed to do was to work with lathes, drills, and tapping machines. We did have to produce a certain amount, however. And because we provided most of the jokes, fun, and laughter among the machine noise and sweat, many of the regular working men would give us a few of their pieces to add to ours to enable us to make our quotas.

It was fun, but it was not easy. Part of the fun was how we got to work in South Ashburnham. We hired a large hay wagon. We all piled onto it, one with a trumpet, another with his violin, and a man with a drum. We sang and played our way to the plant. It's not that we were avoiding the draft this way either — being medical students, we were exempt.

I was also father to a second son, Alfred, born June 26, 1916. Alfred would later attend art schools in Boston and New York and become an art director in advertising firms in New York. His work would become widely recognized, win prizes, and be applauded by *Time Magazine* for a project done by him and his daughter Jeri-Gail; he would work with such Hollywood people as Sophia Loren and Stanley Kubrick, who asked Alfred to design the ads for the movie *Space Odyssey: 2001*.

We knew all too well the seriousness of the war effort and what was happening in Europe. Those left at home had to help as they could. But people also have to know how to smile and have fun, even in the darkest of times. There was a Fourth of July weekend that I remember. We went to Fitchburg and bought firecrackers, frankfurters, and other staples. We tore down some of the old barns and used the wood to prepare a bonfire. We stole some railroad ties too. Then we invited the whole town for that evening. What Fourth of July eve music! What song! We thought we were Yankee Doodle all over again. We marched in front of the town folk musicians, leading them back to their homes, after our grand concert.

I hope you can imagine — upon our return to Boston at the end of the season — our feeling of accomplishment in the war effort, and the thrill of knowing we had earned money enough for school. Another encouraging fact was the knowledge that our work was so satisfactory in this newly acquired trade that we were invited back for the following summer. I like to think that South Ashburnham, a small New England town, perhaps never saw so much life, never had so much fun, and certainly never more warmly welcomed and accepted outsiders as part of the community. In fact, thirty years after we left the factory, my second wife Chloe and I visited the machine shop. Imagine my delight in finding one of the old foremen there — it was a happy reunion! With a twinkle in his eye he said to me, "I never told you of all the spoiled pieces we pulled out of the pond just outside the window." We had thrown them there so we would not look inexperienced.

During the nine months of the third and fourth years of medical school, we spent the morning in clinical practice in various departments. More time had to be devoted to my schooling. Yet, even with all the income from my enterprises, the financial burden was making it difficult to continue. I had to find time to earn more. My stores, of course, were working for me — but I just had to determine where I could give more time. Nights provided the extra hours, and I found a job carrying freight all night long at the Commercial Street freight yards of the Boston and Maine Railroad. But after four months I had to stop because it was impossible for me to stay awake during my school schedule — Boston City Hospital mornings, and afternoon classes and labs — which required my full attention.

The year I was to graduate, the medical requirements for the M.D. degree were changed to include a year of internship. Because of my eighteen months' clinical experience, I gained acceptance for internship as Assistant House Surgeon in the New York Hospital, now part of Cornell Medical Center. It was November 1, 1918, just ten more days until the Armistice. I would have to leave my family behind and dispose of my enterprises. This meant borrowing and seeking financial aid from any source possible. Remember — these were the days when wives did not work outside the home. What helped was that in three and a half months I received a promotion to House Surgeon. As Assistant I had received forty dollars a month; the new position paid sixty dollars, including food, room, and laundry. Because I sent most of the salary home, there was nothing left for visits to Boston. This was the price of the experience and responsibilities associated with House Surgeon. My duties included teaching students from the Bellevue Hospital and supervision of outpatient facilities.

However, I also received living quarters in a beautiful corner suite and had two ambulances at my disposal. Although luxury was no part of my work, I felt as though I was living in such circumstances. We also managed a little fun when not involved with saving lives and restoring people to health. For one thing, during the night hours I learned how to play pinochle, apparently a great New York pastime. Often on Sundays a bunch of us would take the boat to Bear Mountain up the Hudson. The band aboard would play our requests. Or we went to Union Square at times, daringly picking off the metal covers of the barrels as we went along. Or, rolling up our trousers and bandaging our heads, we would march down Broadway in our version of the Spirit of '76. Or when returning from a call with the ambulance without a patient, we would stop in Chinatown or on lower Broadway and play Kelly pool before returning to the hospital. *That* was juvenile delinquency! Neither do I forget how I would take the ambulance clanging away down Second Avenue to Times Square so I could buy the *Boston Post.* Yes, we were serious in a serious profession, and yes, we were boisterous in our spare time. These were ways of relieving the tension.

One of the treasures of my residency is the memory of my immigrant mother coming all the way from Boston to New York for her first opportunity to see her eldest son, the doctor, at work. Her main purpose for the visit, though, was to bring me a gift she thought the well-dressed doctor should have — a fur lined coat with fur collar (this had been an old-world tradition for centuries). This beautiful incident, however, was somewhat marred (an understatement) as a result of that morning's frequent winnings at Kelly pool, the payoff being in wine. Unfortunately, my mother came on a day when I was miserably and flagrantly drunk and sick for the first time in my life, and something never to be repeated. I rarely drank after that, for alcohol affected me too easily. Fortunately my mother, not being a diagnostician, accepted my explanation that I was just innocently sick.

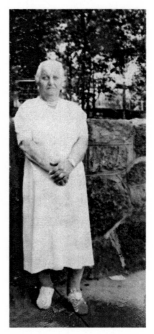

Epta, Morris A. Cohen's mother

I believe these incidents from the internship should be of general interest to the public to let everyone know that even physicians are human beings, that they dedicate themselves to people's welfare, but that they also need relief from life and death situations — through levity, for example, just as do people in other professions, or perhaps more than most. I also tell you these stories because in my work we traveled about and visited the slums, aided the underprivileged, worried and wondered how we could help, forever perplexed by what to do about their health and circumstances. I experienced the lives of these people. They came to influence my future.

What did we observe these people needed most? They needed to regain their health while they remained employed. Even in those pre-inflation times, illness was a catastrophe. The need for alleviating — or preferably, preventing — such total misfortune was silently, often loudly, seeping into me, defining the mission I eventually chose in the practice of medicine. There was, then, not only seriousness in my work but also reflection.

As this was happening, I had responsibilities with which to deal, such as ensuring that we covered all emergencies. In these situations, I was often lenient with interns and students, tempering justice with understanding, because of my awareness of the circumstances in which they worked. Still, I once had the painful duty of firing three interns. Otherwise I would have had to quit my job, according to a notice I received from the Superintendent.

And there was one administrative problem that solved itself. It is the story of the Spanish Count who came to the hospital for four months of training in obstetrics. Never seen without his frock coat, high hat, cane, gloves, or monocle, he was a vision of a perfect aristocrat. Imagine him in these clothes entering an ambulance. Well, one night when all emergency crews were out on calls or working in the hospital, the Count was the only one left on call. Mr. Aloysius, the night clerk, who wore a wig which he would often fish off his head with a hook dangling at the end of a wire, woke me at 3 a.m. to tell me the Count was the only one left, and that he knew the Count was on the premises but that he was not answering his phone. I invited Aloysius to accompany me to the Count's room. There he was, sitting in bed, monocle on, reading and completely unconcerned. I asked him why he did not answer the bell? *"Doctor, I am just too tired."*

Where life saving and efficient operation of the hospital were concerned, and under pressure from the Superintendent to maintain discipline, I could not tolerate this. The very next day the perfect occasion arose to address it. A middle aged Italian-American with torn shirt and wild hair ran into the hospital screaming, "My wife, she go crazy!" His wife had delivered at the hospital and now was evidently experiencing some post-partum maniacal episode. I ordered the clerk to send the Count. The Count appeared dressed for this daytime emergency as I have previously described, except this time he carried his physician's bag. In the other hand were his cane and gloves. About two hours later the second apparition of the day appeared — no cane, gloves, hat or monocle, and an unbuttoned shirt. The Count quit that day.

Now picture me on a typical emergency call on the East Side. There were then "high-rise" living quarters, actually tenements or flats for the low and moderate wage-earners. In describing these living quarters, today's expression "lack of necessities or conveniences" differs little from what it did then. In a typical East Side tenement there was one large room with a partition — formed by wood, parts of furniture or anything else handy — to provide the appearance of separate rooms, hopefully enough material for as many sections as there were family members. Remember that families then were larger than now. The only furniture in those boxed-in mazes was straw — plain straw piled on the floor. That is where we saw the sick and the suffering. To us, these people were just as good as any other human beings; they were deserving, hardworking Americans. In fact, if you look back on the last three quarters of a century, and count the heads of the outstanding Americans who enriched and advanced the life and industry of our country, you will find that many of them grew up in just such an environment as I describe.

Keep this picture in mind. Now imagine the influenza epidemic of 1918, in a large city — an almost certain death among women after delivery. Our pharmacopeia just had not advanced enough to give us either the vaccines or drugs with which to save these lives. After staff consultations, Surgeon-in-Chief Komack decided upon utilizing the entire roof to set up an open field hospital. We did what we could. It will also sound peculiar to physicians and the public of today that we even resorted to bleeding — without success, of course. Most deaths followed lung congestion and pneumonia. It was an insufferable and frustrating time, knowing you are a physician but helpless, watching people suffer and die and being unable to prevent it — recovery depending heavily upon the body's ability to fight the disease.

I was approaching my two thousandth delivery, and my internship would soon end. Most deliveries were in the tenements of the poor. Prior to the end of my time in New York, I received an emergency call from an intern who was having trouble with a breech presentation. Arriving by ambulance, I walked in to find the patient lying on the kitchen table surrounded by about fifty neighbors. The table was in the only open portion of the floor, circled by the usual jumble of materials used for partitions in those so-called apartments. In spite of these surroundings, I completed preparations and set the scene for an operating table with the necessary equipment for the delivery. In that era, we still used chloroform; it was a fast-administering anesthesia, and there was fast recovery from its effects. We needed it for such patients, as you will see.

As soon as the patient was under narcosis, and as I was inserting the forceps for the attempted delivery, the woman's husband suddenly realized his wife was unconscious. He presumed she was dead and rushed at me with a large knife! Intent upon my work, I was unaware of what was happening until in the struggle by the onlookers to restrain him, they jostled me. This awakened me to the added emergency. I suppose had he gotten to me, my death would have been in the line of duty. However, the audience stopped him — and drama or no, I delivered a healthy baby. It was one of the most spectacular public obstetrical demonstrations heard of before modern television. It was also the dramatic finish of my duties.

I now wanted to help to good health the people whose conditions I best knew, those who could pay little or nothing, who perhaps needed care the most. They were people who did not want what politicians presently label the parasitical role of welfare dependency. Somebody had to help these people, and my profession still does. They deserve our aid. It is, however, not only the responsibility of the physicians but of both state and federal governments. If you have emigrated to this country as I did, as I believe many of us have, and if you believe in what you have been taught regarding the people's rights, then surely health care is one of those rights.

It was now time to think of a home for my wife and children, a new practice, and the means for practicing medicine as I intended. To begin practice, though, I would have to take the State Board for licensure. I took a vacation for the first time in my life to study for the examination, which I took in February, 1919. My internship would end May, 1919, when I would experience the momentous occasion of my receipt of the M.D. degree. I then waited for the letter from the State Board of Registration in Medicine — blue if the person passed. When the letter arrived, I asked my little son, Manley, just to tear the corner of the envelope to see the color. It was blue! I could practice medicine.

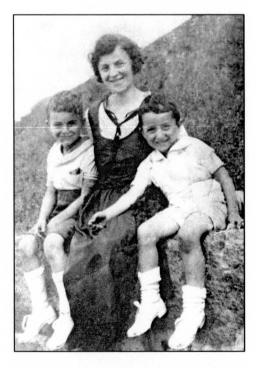

Manley, Anna, Alfred, c. 1919

I do not exactly recall the cash fortune I possessed, but I believe it was just under thirty dollars, when I returned from New York to my family in Boston. How does one start the practice of medicine, buy the necessary medical equipment and furniture, as well as provide for one's family, with thirty dollars! I looked for office space in the area and found a suite of five rooms at 21 McLean Street. An old doctor had just passed away in Chelsea; I bought the entirety of the office furnishings of a man's lifetime of practice for the grand sum of fifty dollars, which an uncle advanced. I *think* I paid it back. Then good friends gave a party and collected a few dollars to buy a table and lamp for the waiting room. The lamp had a lighted base and the bulb in that base lasted about fifteen years, an enduring symbol and reminder of those friends' faith in me.

Around the corner from my new office was St. Joseph's Church. Not too far away, around yet another corner, was my father's new little store on Parkman Street. Nearby also at the time was the Boston Lying-in Hospital. With preparations for practice complete, in spite of the hospital being where it was, I still believed my first consideration for care should be the people of Boston's West End who had given me the vision of my lifetime's work.

Obstetrics meant a large practice in those days because families were large, and despite hospitals, most deliveries were at home. My reputation, because of my New York experience, traveled ahead of me by word of mouth; parents, friends, relatives, and neighbors spread the word. It was not too long before my practice was lively. Before ten months had passed, I had paid for a Ford automobile. That was a real thrill!

My brother Alfred told me the story of this Ford. One morning after having worked most of the night, my father tried to sleep in, but the noise of an automobile awakened him. Angrily he went to the window and bellowed, "Will you get that car out of here!" The person or people obeyed, and drove off — in my father's new Ford.

— Richard S. Cohen

My obstetrical reputation I thought, one day, had spread a little too far when my father's sister sent the entire family to plead with me to take her case and deliver her at home in Chelsea. She was in great difficulty, in danger of either a too-early delivery or unintended abortion. She hesitated to ask me directly to take her case and instead sent massive persuasion. The family was convinced that my experience must be placed at her disposal to ensure preservation of the child's life. You are aware that I owed a lot, one way or another, to my family — including the uncle who had me arrested as a horse thief. They had been good to me through the years, and despite quarrels there remained a closeness of family. Although physicians do not normally treat close relatives, I yielded, and delivered my aunt of a normal girl.

In a relatively short time, I was now supporting my family by the practice of medicine. An addition to the family arrived at this time, our third son, George, born January 16, 1920 (now a successful practicing optometrist who contributes his time evenings with me at the Clinic).

CHAPTER THREE:
ESTABLISHMENT, AGAINST ODDS

By 1920, only a year after I started the practice of medicine, a new era began unfolding in medicine, that of specialization. There was urgent need for additional clinical training for physicians to fill one of those new fields, physical and rehabilitation medicine. Its orientation was for working people liable to injury and disablement in the country's growing industrial and manufacturing companies. I believed this field was precisely the means by which I could best serve the laboring class I knew. Therefore, in spite of the additional economic stress on the support of my family, I enrolled in training at the Boston City Hospital.

It was a new field, but few physicians were as yet interested in practicing this specialty. The few who were, formed a society named The New England Society of Physical Medicine. In 1925, I became treasurer of this society. In that same year we held the first scientific clinical session at the then Copley Plaza Hotel in Boston. I had charge of the arrangements for the industrial exhibits display, as well as of program arrangements for scientific papers. It was also my first scientific presentation at a medical convention. My paper, "Physical Measures in Acute Trauma," was published afterwards in the *American Journal of Surgery* in early 1926. The presentation was a scientific clinical discussion of practices and results in this new field of therapy for working people hurt or disabled in industry.

Because we were successful with the reduction of the period of disability and rehabilitation related to industrial injuries, we were able to receive a larger number of patient referrals through Workmen's Compensation, from employers and from insurance companies such as Liberty Mutual and American

Mutual. Such clinical rehabilitation results would lead to the establishment of physical medicine rehabilitation clinics. This was also a part of the seed for the Boston Evening Clinic that I started later. The new field also progressed, becoming well established and well understood because of its wide application and results. It therefore necessitated the training of more doctors for practice in this specialty. This was actually the birth of industrial medicine as we know it today.

There was still another reason that the clinic I envisioned became a necessity. Consider that under the State Workmen's Compensation Law, workers only received fourteen to sixteen dollars per week from insurance while they were out of work as a result of industrial injuries and disease. Despite the fact that the period of disability was considerably reduced because of the new clinical rehabilitation approach, we began to take notice of the disastrous effect upon workers and their families when illness reduced weekly pay to this new minimum compensation. As long as workers needed care, which often meant frequent visits to morning or day clinics over an extended period of time, obviously the person could not return to work and to a regular salary. Further, long waiting hours at the daytime clinics precluded work on the day of the clinic visit. An extensive series of visits would very likely jeopardize the job. This deprived families of the necessities of life during convalescence, especially in cases of prolonged absence from work, and even afterward. This economic deprivation had tragic consequences to family life: the unavailability of clinic attention during other than daytime working hours caused the patient to stay away from hospitals until desperately ill.

Therefore, physicians could not ignore or avoid becoming involved in the practical problems faced by the moderate-to low-income workers. It became not only a medical problem but a moral and ethical question as well. If the person was to be helped, the *whole* situation must be studied — the person's health care issue needed to be structured around *anticipated* problems. From what we in my specialty observed, the dilemma could not be solved by the existing medical institutions and their completely unrealistic provisions for workers' care. After all, illness can be prolonged or worsened by unnecessary fears of lengthy absences from work. Clinic hours set to accommodate the physician's convenience rather than that of the patient constituted a punishing burden on those who were ill. In most cases, one visit incurred the loss of a day's pay, in addition to possible hospital costs. Certainly such care is not therapeutic and *does not promote recovery, but contributes to situational pathology.*

Might not the same be said today as the world changes to more highly technical skills? With more and more people entering the workforce at different levels, and thus with more and more families affected by that workforce, the tensions increase regarding absence from work because of health concerns, including fear over ability to pay. These are facts we must face as a society, not only as physicians.

Thus it was — because no one was considering the problem of care for the low- to moderately-paid worker — that the period between 1923 and 1927 became a planning period for the Boston Evening Clinic, originally called the Boston Reconstruction Clinic. Ways needed to be developed to establish the Clinic on a firm basis. Part of that basis was keeping current with advancements in physical medicine as they began to appear through the contributions of leaders in the specialty, most of whom were concentrated in Boston and New York. It was therefore necessary for me to arrange visits to observe and to work with these men from time to time, generally for one- or two-week periods. Yet, there would be more personal decisions necessitated.

I had an associate for a while in the new venture, Dr. Louis Feldman, who had also been practicing in the West End and who had joined me in training at the Boston City Hospital. With him, we took up quarters for the new specialty in industrial medicine, a six-room, fully equipped suite at 360 Commonwealth Avenue in Boston. We hoped that such a clinic would attract patients we wanted to help by being an institution established specifically for them, a place where the people would feel they had a *right* to be, rather than believing they were either the afterthought or a burden.

It was also necessary to assure the appropriate equipment and staff. The equipment for this new practice, today termed "industrial medicine," was quite expensive: it included faradic and galvanic machines for the regeneration of nerve tissue, sinusoidal machines, whirlpool baths, and an x-ray machine to help diagnose injuries. How was all this equipment purchased? I really cannot now recall all the financial arrangements of that time; all I can say is that it was done. I do know that I established myself in that practice, part of which was referral by other physicians, part by insurance companies, part by various industries.

The first employee groups I took were the then growing Checker Taxi and Town Taxi Companies, for which I performed pre-employment examinations and treatment of injured employees. I still care for the employees of these two companies after forty-four years.

As for the first medical staff of the Reconstruction Clinic, the physicians served without compensation. They did benefit, of course, from industrial accident cases referred by insurance companies or employers, not to the Clinic but to themselves. On the roster of these dedicated physicians were: Dr. Leroy R. G.

Crandon, surgery; Dr. Irving Walker, surgery; Dr. Frederick Cotton, consultant in orthopedics; Dr. Augustus Thorndike, consultant in skin diseases; Dr. William D. Wheeler, skin diseases; Dr. David Butler, nose and throat; and Drs. Maurice A. Lesser, Evelyn G. Mitchell, and Harry Golden.

Our first trial of evening clinic hours was so successful in restoring the well-being of so many workers and their families that the Clinic progressed from a plan to a demonstration for serving the health care underclass. We were now helping people I consider courageous, those who despite disability and, too often, chronic discomfort and pain, resolutely stayed on the job to support their families and continued as productive members of society.

1927, then, was the beginning of the Reconstruction Evening Clinic. Doctors began referring patients for evening treatment. Many patients heard from others about the convenient hours after work and the low cost, and began coming in such numbers that before long you could say *we had bitten off more than we could chew.* During the first year the attendance increased from twenty-five to over three thousand five hundred; doctors were added to keep pace with these numbers.

The Evening Clinic hours began to be well known to the medical world and its institutions. The response spread quickly from the patients, for whose neglected needs our services had been planned. Gradually, too, we found ourselves doing the greater portion of our work for partial payments or for free. Therefore, despite the contributed time of doctors and technicians, by the end of that first year there was a substantial deficit. My personal income would have to erase the debt. This added to my personal financial problems. Yet, the enormous need for the Clinic and the beneficial results of its work left me with no other alternative.

There also began to be repercussions at home. It must be imagined that a husband with a mission was surely someone of whom to be proud; however it would be an unusual wife indeed who could weather with complete stoicism the loneliness due to a frequently absent husband, as well as a dwindling of financial support and the resulting sacrifices for wife, household, and children. More on the outcome of all this later in the story.

— Richard S. Cohen

Lacking financial support and requiring increased staff, we initiated three ventures to provide the Clinic with paramedical help, as well as with additional physicians, all of whom could eventually assist in the Clinic. The plan included:

1. — Courses, without cost, of lectures and clinical training in the new field of physical and rehabilitation medicine.

2. — A training school for physical therapy technicians who would assist in treatment without pay while in training, but who learned while assisting, in much the same way as do newly graduated medical students who enter internship (though today they are paid substantially more than I received when training). Like the physical training courses, the schooling included lectures and related physics, chemistry, anatomy, physiology, some pathology, and the theory and clinical aspects of physical therapy measures that included traction, massage and manipulation, and therapeutic exercises for rehabilitation. (Such training may sound commonplace today, and think of how much of this one now sees on television, but not so in 1927.)

3. — A laboratory school. The laboratory, a vital part of the Clinic, was rapidly expanding; therefore I made the decision

that we should train our own technicians. In fact, one of our graduates of thirty years ago, Mabel Bing You, still works in our laboratory today.

Not only was the Clinic growing in attendance and in the training delivered, but I also recognized the need for increasing my own knowledge in industrial and rehabilitative medicine in order to assure fulfillment of my purposes for the Clinic. I could make only one decision, that being to abandon much of my own medical practice to acquire the necessary additional training. I went to Dr. Frank B. Granger, Chief of the Department of Physical Medicine and Rehabilitation at Boston City Hospital and told him of my willingness to give time and training in that department. I imagine it was my eagerness for service that led him to accept me as a visiting assistant for training and practice in the Department. I also spent some time with Dr. Ellsworth in the X-Ray Department of the hospital. Naturally, my attendance at the hospital five mornings a week devastated my daytime earnings. To compensate, I added more night calls.

After this training at the Boston City Hospital, I took time to visit the Reconstruction Hospital in New York where rehabilitation, then labeled reconstruction, was taught to physician trainees. I spent some time there in clinical observation and took advanced courses with, among others, Dr. William Benham Snow, the leader in the field. Having received this additional learning, I made the decision to abandon general practice entirely. This did not mean I could ignore the necessity to earn for the support of my family, so I took on a job as police surgeon for Station 16, another for the Boxing Commission two or three evenings a week, and a third making calls to hotel patrons as hotel physician. I was back at work — hard work — earning weekly wages again. It was not an unbearable burden, however, because the Clinic was proving to be a success.

But by 1928 — the year of the birth of our fourth son, Richard — the opposition of the medical establishment became more apparent. In this year our colleague Dr. Simon Cox, who was also a member of the Massachusetts Medical Society, received an order to appear before the Committee of Ethics and Discipline. (Dr. Cox was a Harvard Medical School classmate of Dr. David Cheever. To the former I shall pay special attention in the history of the Clinic. During this particular period, he served as Superintendent of the Clinic, and I as Medical Director, neither of us receiving any salary. Dr. Cox had his own income from individual institutional practice.) The Committee asked Dr. Cox for information about the Clinic, its organization, its purpose. More revealing was the question, "Why do you persist when the Society has so many complaints about the Clinic from so many doctors?"

Following upon this, I, too, received an order to appear. They asked the same questions, made the same criticism. The worst affront, however, was the suggestion that we were using our patients for personal profit. I asked how anyone could imagine there was financial gain when we received only fifty cents for every dollar expended in the operation of the Clinic!

Dissatisfied, the Committee continued its investigation indirectly. And shortly after my appearance, I learned that some institutions interrogated members of their staffs who also helped at the Clinic. Those institutions asked for information about the Clinic and the reasons why those physicians served on the Clinic staff. It is not easy for me, even at this late date, to relate that several of these institutions then told some members of our staff to make a choice either to serve on their staffs or the Clinic's. That was an awful choice to present to a doctor who needs hospital affiliation in order to engage in the practice of medicine. Furthermore, seldom could a physician socially, economically, professionally, or in any other way pursue the practice of medicine without membership in the Medical Society. It is the first question asked by institutions in organized medicine, whether for inquiries regarding a physician's qualification, for association with the institution, or just for admission to their scientific sessions. There were some rebels, however, who continued to serve us under this threat.

Membership is now optional in a Medical Society. This information is from Morris Cohen's grandson, Mylan C. Cohen, MD., M.P.H., President of the American Society of Nuclear Cardiologists in 2010 and a partner in Maine Cardiology Associates, Portland, Maine.

— Richard S. Cohen

When 1929 came, it was all too clear I personally would have to continue to support the Reconstruction Evening Clinic. I often had to borrow to pay the Clinic bills. Needless to say, my family was sometimes deprived of necessities, and of course we did not even think of luxuries.

Despite economic problems, the spectacular good of the evening clinic hours for those who had no choice but to stay on the job, and for those who could pay but little or nothing for medical care, had now been incontrovertibly demonstrated. The need which I had seen was validated. The reason for our existence could no longer be rationalized or wished away by the medical community.

There was, however, the continuing nagging question of how to continue care for the hundreds of people sent to us or who came on their own with so little funds. I consulted with an attorney, Joseph Brettler, who advised me that to continue giving service with inadequate compensation, it would be necessary to organize the Clinic as a public charity, in order to ask others for financial help.

It would take seven citizens to form the corporation. The persons who would be added to the group were: Alice Stone Blackwell, Pitt W. Danforth, Frank Sawyer, Joseph Brettler, and Joseph Brin, my old newsboy friend. On November 27, 1929, we petitioned the Department of Public Welfare for a charter. The Commissioner was Ralph Conant, who after a public hearing had discretion to grant the charter.

I already knew there was cooperation from and interest in the Clinic's work from eminent laypeople, clergy, and other citizens who were aware of the Clinic's value and the need for such an institution. At this time, too, the press interviewed Evelyn G. Mitchell, a member of the Clinic staff. It was obvious from this support and the interest of the press, that the public was aware of a new idea and effort, a different way of helping the modest wage earner and the poor while supporting or encouraging appreciation of individual worth.

My father had a hunting dog named Dick. Perhaps I was named after the dog. Anyhow, at the age of two or three, I slept in a crib in my folks' bedroom, and the dog slept under my crib, often howling and scaring me. I would stand up and scream in fear.

Off this room, my parents' bedroom, was an alcove with another door beyond which was my father's home office. In a window of our living room was a black and white sign with the name, Morris A. Cohen, M.D. I remember knowing of the home office and what my father's profession was by the time I was four, especially on the day a janitor came to the back door, begging to see the doctor. He had a fishing lure with what seemed to me a large hook stuck deeply in his thumb. My mother told him the doctor was not at home but that the man should come with her. I followed, and in that home medical room, I watched her gently take his hand, working at the hook until she freed the man of the lure. She cleaned the wound and bandaged it.

My mother, though I did not know it then, had started to study nursing. She later gave this up, perhaps to have another child, or in order to devote her time to her voice lessons.

— Richard S. Cohen

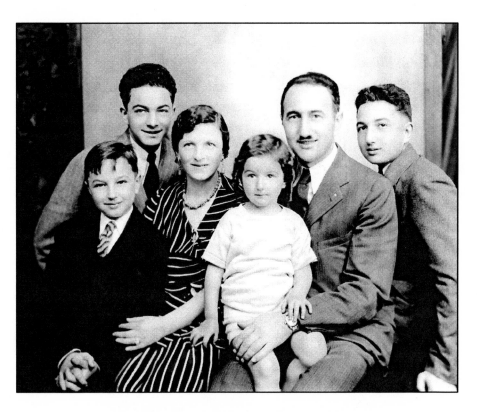

The Family, c. 1931: from left to right—
George, Manley, Anna, Richard, Morris, Alfred

CHAPTER FOUR: ADVERSITY AND CHARTER

It never occurred to me, when we petitioned for the charter, that any person would object or try to prevent such an indispensable nonprofit public health service, other than (possibly) some established medical institution. I did not anticipate the assault that came. The experience was reminiscent of my father confronting the rockbound soil of Canada that was un-tillable. He was alone, facing a hostile wilderness, just as I now was. I believed, however, that my training and membership in the profession would allow me to overcome unforeseen problems. As time passed, though, the shots and barrages became a bombardment.

At first I refused to believe that the cannonade came from my own profession. I was prepared to grapple with physical and financial obstacles but not the unanticipated barriers of disapproval from doctors sworn to the same oath as I upon becoming physicians, from the medical establishment, and from institutions representing the public welfare and whose duty it was to serve the people. I found it totally incomprehensible! Living in a large city, having practiced in that city, I was, it became apparent, as ingenuous and unsophisticated as a country boy when it came to the ways of organized medicine. I was reluctant to accept that individuals and organizations we believe to be devoted to serving one's fellow humans should emerge as antagonists. It was particularly hard because earlier, these people and institutions, including the Chamber of Commerce and the *New England Journal of Medicine*, professed sympathy and gave encouragement.

To see my dream established, hard work was an easy price tag compared to the obstacles — the protests, opposition, and challenges from the various quarters of my profession. Laboring when I was younger to lift goods from the ground to a freight car, in retrospect, seemed much easier than the load caused by the protests against the Clinic. Worse yet, after submission of the petition for the charter, we discovered that many who hoped to prevent approval advised Mr. Conant not to grant the charter. When repeatedly asked the reason for the delay, Mr. Conant parried by asking for further information.

In the face of such continued opposition, we believed that petitioning for a charter and forming the Clinic as a public charity, an organization responsible to the Department of Public Welfare and administered by a body of citizens, would quell the outcry and allow us to deliver our work free of the misconceptions fostered about the organization.

As we approached the end of 1929, I continued in private referred practice in the new specialty field, industrial medicine. The Clinic, now located on a nine-room floor at 366 Commonwealth Avenue, was functioning with a well organized staff. Two training schools furnished us with clinical aides. Yet, we still encountered more and more hostility and harassment from doctors, medical societies and institutions, and social service agencies. It was bewildering. We were unremittingly distracted by those who refused to believe our factual presentations. In fact, the complaints were so intrusive that we had to increase our efforts just to keep our attention focused on our work. These attacks consumed too much of our time. More unfortunately, the continuous effort needed in order to explain and defend our mission and activities to the misinformed were all to no avail. The consequence to me of these diversions of effort was that the opposition forced me to neglect my practice, and this cost me income which was the lifeblood of the Clinic, of which I was still the major sustaining support of its operation.

An upheaval of vociferous, open antagonism had arisen within the entire social service-medical community. It was totally beyond our understanding. I appealed to friends, to authorities, and to representatives of various institutions in order to discover the reasons for the outcries, for I believed it was within my power to correct the misconceptions.

Perhaps the most disheartening day of my life, during this period, was when Dr. Leroy R.G. Crandon called me to his office to tell me that the opposition to the Clinic by the medical world was too great for him to continue. Crandon, Chief of Surgery at the Boston City Hospital and Professor of Surgery at Harvard Medical School, was one of my dearest friends and a trusted advisor. That day he told me it would be impossible to overcome this antagonism and to continue with this valuable work. Advised unequivocally to do so, he handed me his resignation from the staff. He then said that for my family's welfare and to preserve my personal practice of medicine, I should close the Clinic. Acting upon advice he had received, he handed me a stamped envelope and a piece of his personal stationery, addressed to Dr. David Cheever of the Massachusetts Medical Society. The purpose of this action was to urge me without delay to notify Dr. Cheever that I would close the Clinic.

Were we not helping people whose human and physical circumstances had been largely ignored? There was no other part pay/free *evening* clinic to safeguard blue collar people's daytime work hours, their paychecks, and the support of their families, from ruinous medical expense! What the Medical Society demanded of me was completely illogical. Had we not inaugurated an immeasurably valuable new remedy for a serious public health situation?

Despite my convictions and shaken by Dr. Crandon's advice,

I did write the letter to Dr. Cheever. Instead of mailing it, however, I called together some of the medical staff to tell them of the interview with Crandon. At the meeting were Drs. William D. Wheeler, Maurice A Lesser, David Butler, Harry Golden, Evelyn Mitchell, and Simon Cox. When I recounted my session with Crandon, they confronted me: "How do you dare? Isn't this a decision to be made with others?" Dr. Butler tore the letter from my hand while telling me, "Morris Cohen, you are not going to do it!" He ripped the letter into pieces. All I had left in my hand was that memorable Cheever envelope. Our work would not cease. The Clinic would not close.

Discouraging days, exhausting days of tension, anxiety in the midst of work, continual financial stress, and family concerns should have overwhelmed me. There was, however, this kind of continued commitment of the medical staff that sustained me. Increasingly under pressure themselves from staff associates elsewhere, from institutions, and from the Medical Society that they resign, some had to — but many believed steadfastly enough in the work to say, "No!" Keep in mind, too, that the medical staff served without pay and even made financial contributions to help offset the deficit. What emerges clearly from that uncertain period is my memory of devoted physicians who had nothing to gain and who risked so much. Simply put, they were receiving the same intangible — rather than actual — compensation intrinsic in this new concept of care for the helpless. This was the way we kept the evening clinic concept alive.

It was not very long before I was again called to appear before the Committee of Ethics and Discipline. On the morning of my appearance, Dr. Crandon's nurse, Miss Durling, brought me a note from Dr. Crandon telling me he had retracted his resignation from the Clinic staff and would continue to serve! He was well aware of what was happening from

43

information I gave when I frequently visited his home to treat Mrs. Crandon's mother.

At the Committee meeting, its members told me, "Doctors will resign from the Clinic. Dr. Crandon already has." How, I wondered, did they know that? They asked, "How do you intend to continue?" I had no alternative but to produce, to their astonishment, the letter Dr. Crandon had sent that very morning.

Once again I asked the Committee for a decision, whether — and why — they continued to see us as engaged in unethical practices. I asked what, exactly, were their objections? And, "What is your advice?" The reply was silence. Then, "No findings." The meeting ended. It was a terribly depressing, ominous cloud under which to work, for the Committee affected the entire operation of the Clinic, support of which still depended upon a continually threatened medical staff.

These appalling problems of the early years of the Clinic were the most challenging. I could not be swayed from serving those who were unquestionably in need of health care. It was a time when no other institution offered comprehensive medical care, "Group Practice," such as is now nationally advertised and practiced. I believe, if you look through medical literature and history, you will find that ours was the beginning of group practice for the benefit of the moderate/low wage worker and is exactly parallel with the quality offered by private group practice to those who can pay full fees.

It is important to realize that this account was written before the advent of HMOs and the widespread practice of relying on insurance companies for partial payment of health services, before President Johnson's later introduction of Medicare and Medicaid, and before today's debate regarding fee-for-service, prescription drugs, and the panoply of delivery problems which exist.

— *Richard S. Cohen*

That the Clinic continued to operate without visible means of support was also a source of consternation to the medical establishment. Again I received a letter, this time to appear before the Committee of Ethics and Discipline of the Massachusetts Medical Society. The Committee's head was Dr. L.C. Smith of Brockton. It was to be a crucial and consequential meeting, for Dr. Smith asked me, "How do you propose to conduct such part pay/free medical service when large institutions are running deficits of hundreds of thousands of dollars in supplying such services daytimes?" Admittedly he was plain spoken. "How do you, Dr. Morris Cohen, propose to do such a thing in light of your financial circumstances?"

The members of the Committee seemed very well informed regarding all conditions of the operation of the Clinic. It was formidable facing this inquisition, answering such questions. There was only one way. I replied, in substance, *"Dr. Smith and Gentlemen of the Committee: I was brought up in the very slums of this city among these people whose needs and wants I know and am trying to relieve. I lived in the cellars and dark alleys of those slums."*

I then told the story you have so far read, of how I received my education and prepared to become a doctor who would serve these very people. I described how what I was doing became my ideal for the practice of medicine. I stated that if that day or the next, or any other day they knew of one hundred or two hundred or more of these people I was trying to help who were not receiving health care, they should send them to the Clinic. We would take care of them.

Somehow, at last, my statements at this meeting carried enough conviction to change minds. We received a letter, signed by the then president, Dr. John M. Birnie, which read in part, *"The high altruistic and charitable purposes that animate those who conduct the Clinic with which you are associated should be a source of satisfaction to all those who have the best interest of your profession at heart."*

We had finally received the judgment we wanted! It was a happy day indeed when that letter arrived. It was confirmation — in fact, vindication — of what we were doing, recognition of our cause. The Medical Society rekindled our resolve. Now that our sincerity of purpose received acknowledgment, I could look forward, hopefully, to the certainty of being able to carry on the work. It was a joyous staff meeting at which I read this document.

We now felt that the way was cleared, and our Clinic approved, so that Mr. Conant, Commissioner of Public Welfare, would be influenced to use his discretionary power to grant us the charter. That was not to be soon or easy, however, despite the kindness of then Governor Allen, who wrote me at the time that he had personally approached Mr. Conant. Even the Governor could not convince Mr. Conant to change his mind or grant the charter! Our struggle was to continue.

We now needed to bring the struggle with Mr. Conant to resolution, and legal counsel told me that there was a way — to overcome what appeared to be wrongly applied discretionary power, we would have to show that Conant ignored evidence that our work was an ethically administered charity designed to remedy an ignored medical need, and that our medical aid to the underprivileged constituted unique benefits to this neglected group. The charter should then be granted by a special act of the legislature.

Through the efforts of men such as Philip Markley, Ernest Dean, William Jones and other friends from the legislature, a bill appeared in 1932. Its presentation had to be before the Public Welfare Committee of the House, my good friend Mr. Jones being the Chairman. It was necessary to hold a public meeting because of much opposition from various sources and agencies. Because of overcrowding, there was an adjournment to allow a move to Gardner Auditorium, a larger hall. What made the day so much more historic is the memory of Alice Stone Blackwell, niece of Elizabeth Stone, the first female physician in the country. Ms. Blackwell early befriended the Clinic, in keeping with her lifelong involvement in social movements. Ill on the day of the hearing, she nevertheless called me that morning to say that she insisted on attending the meeting and speaking for the Clinic. "All you need to do, Morris," she said, "is to bring a pillow and blanket for me." That is how she went to this meeting, attended by about 500 others.

Mr. Conant appeared this day before the Committee's executive session and demanded, "Under what circumstances do the members of the Committee believe they can make laws of the Commonwealth under which I am given such discretionary powers?" With such admonishment, some members of the Committee became hesitant, halting action at that meeting on the proposed bill.

This was about the middle of May, 1932. The following week, at a meeting of the Public Welfare Committee, Mr. Jones again brought up the bill for discussion. It passed with recommendation for action by the full House, May 15, 1932. The Bill passed through a first reading in the morning and a second reading in the afternoon.

Panic then let loose in the State House on the part of the Public Welfare Department. Mr. Conant and others appeared in

Representative Ernest Dean's office and in the Speaker's office. Mr. Conant confronted them with the opposition of various health and welfare agencies, as well as prominent private citizens, doctors, and medical societies to granting the charter to the Clinic.

The next morning, May 16, I received a call from Speaker Leverett Saltonstall, with whom I was on friendly terms, who requested I appear in his office June 16. I asked Ernest Dean to accompany me, as I was not experienced in politics.

When we met, Mr. Saltonstall explained that the strong opposition to the bill made the passage of it an impossible task. I vividly recall Mr. Dean firmly saying to Mr. Saltonstall: "Mr. Speaker, this is *wrong!* All that these people are trying to do is to do good. They are not asking for compensatory reward. They just want to serve, to help. What's wrong with that?" He paused, and then continued, "Mr. Speaker, we shall pass this legislation in THIS legislature, because such use of discretionary power under any legal phase should not be tolerated."

Saltonstall told me he would speak to Mr. Conant to see whether it would be possible to arrive at some compromise. If this would not satisfy Conant, Mr. Saltonstall would do all he could to help. He was interested in what we were doing. From this point on, what I can say about Mr. Saltonstall's service to the community, the state, and the country, is that it was beneficial in many ways other than financial. I strongly treasure his expressions of encouragement and sympathy for our work.

That June 16, there was a short morning session of the House. Not having time to finish our conversation prior to the short Bunker Hill Day pre-holiday session, Mr. Saltonstall invited me to come to the House and to sit there during the session so that afterwards we could continue our conversation. Then, June 19, I received a call from him that he had made an appointment for the members of our Board to meet in Mr. Conant's office to discuss the problem.

That morning, at about eleven a.m., our Board members — Mr. Danforth, Mr. Brettler, Miss Blackwell, Mr. Jonsson, Mr. Brin, and I — after lengthy discussion with Mr. Conant, were finally told that he was seriously considering granting the charter, that if we would hold a special meeting and elect Mr. Danforth President, Mr. Sawyer Treasurer, and Mr. Brin Secretary and present such results to him, he would act favorably. I asked Mr. Conant if he had any objection if we retired immediately to the hall. He appeared stunned by such prompt action. We held our special meeting outside his office in the State House corridor and returned in less than ten minutes. Satisfied, Mr. Conant said he would grant the charter. We told him the charter should be retroactive to the date of application, November 27, 1929, because taxes had accrued since our petition.

On June 23, Mr. Brin, now Secretary of the Board and who was doing special work for Frederick W. Cook, Secretary of State, called to tell me the charter was ready in Mr. Cook's office; and that the latter, knowing of the difficulties we had overcome, thought it would be nice to take a photographer with me to record the charter granting. The picture now hangs in my office.

Ironically, just the previous day, Frank Sawyer called me to inquire whether we had received the charter, because he had heard that one or more of the large fundraising agencies or institutions was presenting new opposition. For the moment, however, enemies mattered little. It was a day of jubilation. We celebrated!

Meanwhile, my family also grew with the birth of our fifth child, a daughter, Selma, who joined the group of children, all of whom have brought me joy as a father.

After all the years of boys, Selma Marilyn was born. When my father took us to the hospital to see my new sister, my first remark was, "Her head looks like a football." But Selma grew into a beautiful blonde blue-eyed child. Later she studied voice and piano. In later years she thought of becoming a nurse, a profession she greatly admires. If you asked her today, she would tell you she should have become a nurse because of the caring and marvelous work they perform. She also admires my father for the work he did in bringing the Clinic to life. In her eyes, the Clinic is part of our lives.

— Richard S. Cohen

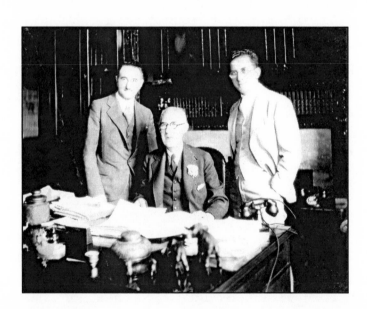

Granting of the Clinic Charter — taken June 23, 1932. From left to right: Morris A. Cohen; Frederick W. Cook, Massachusetts Secretary of State; Mr. Joseph Brin, Secretary of the Clinic Board

A word about the home front during these years. When I was young, the Clinic was not a dominant element in my life — I was largely unaware of any pressure or stress. To my young eyes, all was harmony. My mother, Anna Shain Cohen, had a magnificent voice and managed to attend the New England Conservatory for a couple of years and then took private singing lessons from one of Boston's outstanding voice teachers. Our house was filled with music, which everyone loved and by which we were all influenced: Manley played the violin and was a singer in the Harvard Glee Club, Alfred was a natural at the piano, George was a radio singer at twelve, and Selma, when old enough, was taught voice, acting, and piano. Even my dad played the harmonica quite well. I just listened and learned. I can also remember my mother singing to me so I would fall asleep: "Climb upon my knee sonny boy / Though you're only three, sonny boy . . ."

My mother also managed to take advantage of her place in the community that rose from my father's profession. She knew any number of doctors' wives and other women. She became known to some extent, I imagine, because of her voice. She appeared in musicals, such as playing Buttercup in "The Pirates of Penzance." She also sang in a choir. I can remember looking down from a balcony in either the then Copley Plaza or the Statler when she was in rehearsal with the choir, in which she was a lead voice. She must have been at least partly acknowledged as prominent throughout the Boston area, for after a shipwreck during a trip with Selma and me, a large photo of her face — the only one on the front page — appeared in one of the Boston papers. I discovered this much later while going through microfilm one day while doing research at a university at which I worked. It must be remembered that women in that day did not have the freedom they have today. But she did manage to do much of what she wanted, largely because she had help at home — she had maids, and a nanny, a Mrs. Gannon, whom I loved dearly as a second mother, and who was so kind to me. However my real mother was undisputed head of the house — but in family matters only.

Music may have filled the house, but harmony within was increasingly crowded out by the Clinic and its conflicts, and by lack of unity — suppressed, at least when I was around — between my mother and father. I was also as yet unaware of my father's absences from home growing more frequent. I knew about the Clinic at this time, because of my father's hours. What I did not know about was the widening gap between my parents and that it, also, kept him away. It was obvious he was a physician and that because of his hours, he needed rest when he came home. However, I did hear the word "clinic." When I was 5 or 6, I realized there was a clinic and that my father also had a private practice. What I did not find out until later was that he used money from his private practice to ensure that the Clinic could remain open.

It was when I was about six years of age that I had pneumonia and whooping cough. My father, as I recall, was often by my bedside to help as he could and to ensure I was progressing. Those were the days without antibiotics. In fact, about two years later, a cousin died from meningitis because of the lack of treatment medication. My father also tried to help there. It was of no use, of course. People often hear or are aware that doctors do not treat their own families. However, when there was a disease other than a cold, my father was always there.

— Richard S. Cohen

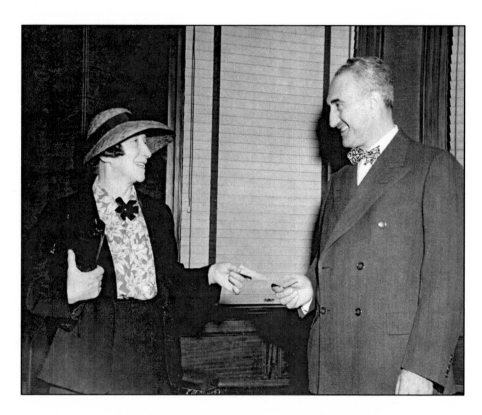

*A grateful patient presents a Christmas check
to the Medical Director, Morris A. Cohen*

CHAPTER FIVE: LIES AND OMISSIONS

On the day I presented the Charter to the trustees, I also gave an inventory of our equipment, including furniture, x-ray, physical therapy apparatus, laboratory, surgical instruments, and drugs, including all other materials used in the operation of the Clinic.

There was also the matter of funds for continuing our work. I had just received a check for two thousand dollars, made out in full to the Clinic, from an insurance company as settlement for my son George who received a fractured skull when an automobile veered onto the sidewalk on which he was walking. The trustees contributed five hundred dollars more at this meeting. Moreover, ninety percent of the staff served without pay, including me as Medical Director. There was paid clerk help, accounting for the other ten percent.

So with this accounting, we now began to operate as a public charity under the supervision of the State Departments of Public Welfare, Public Health, and the Attorney General's Office. These entities supervised operation of all legally chartered charities in the Commonwealth.

Yet, as amateurs in charitable work, and apart from occasional but welcome small gifts from grateful patients, we did not receive much financial aid. I still had to contribute most of my private practice income. Appallingly, also, we gradually became aware of continued antagonism in the fundraising arena. It became glaringly apparent that potential contributors were receiving advice not to give. It was an almost unbelievable aggression against the Clinic. During the years since starting, we had to answer too frequently to criticism and to face antagonism. The attempts to prevent operation of the

Clinic continued. Disparagement pervaded all avenues of charitable funding organizations. We were ostracized, generally unacknowledged as a charitable trust. This attitude by established medical, charitable, and social service agencies, including the Chamber of Commerce, never stopped. No friendly doors opened to us. Not one of us could discover why. This established hostile attitude was a severe, destructive stumbling block to our attempts to obtain public financial support. This attitude toward the Clinic was heartbreaking and made it more difficult to operate. All the while our clinical work occurred with resounding success, never a complaint regarding the quality of clinical practice.

Upon the granting of the charter, the trustees, the staff, and all others interested in the Clinic believed that acceptance would be assured by recognition by the state authorities that the institution was charitable and was duplicating that of no other medical or social service agency. That was not to be for many years to come. For now, it did not matter that in accordance with institutional staff ethical procedures we had on file staff doctors' applications, stating qualifications and branch of medicine. And, at the request of the Department of Public Welfare, we had to ask each staff doctor to state that he or she was serving on the Clinic staff. We transmitted these statements to Mr. Conant, the Commissioner of Public Welfare.

There were other problems, in addition to economic obstruction. During the four years prior to the charter being granted, we conducted training, free of charge, for physicians in the new field of physical medicine and laboratory technique. We carried announcements in the *Massachusetts Medical Society Journal*. The Society's journal would not carry any notice unless there was evidence that we conformed to the code of ethics and that all teaching members be members of the Society. I was a member at that time, as were all the doctors on the staff. But about a year after the granting of the charter, without explanation, more than fifteen doctors suddenly resigned!

Stunned by the enormity of this disaster and lacking any information regarding the calamity, I was ignorant regarding the cause until the next morning. Then one of the most loyal members asked to come see me to show me a very important communication which puzzled him and left him at loss for the proper action. He brought me a communication from Dr. Walter Bowers, editor of the *New England Journal of Medicine*, the publication of the Massachusetts Medical Society, stating that the Clinic recently applied for advertising and asking that the staff member write and tell Dr. Bowers his position at the Clinic, what his work was, and whether he received compensation. The staff reaction was not surprising, considering that the letter from the official journal of the medical society stated that the Clinic had "applied for advertising."

The staff physicians had received this communication in error. The truth was that the Clinic's *announcement* had been routinely inserted in the *Journal* during the previous two to three years. The staff physicians made a logical inference, implied by the letter, that our announcement was a new, and unethical, commercial advertisement. Therefore they resigned, fearing the wrath of the Massachusetts Medical Society's Committee on Ethics and Discipline.

This was a new catastrophe that caused me panic. I did not know what to do about the patients who would come as usual. There had already occurred an increase of visits, both with and without referral from physicians, health, welfare, and social agencies, and because of our reputation for service for fifty cents or nothing. It had not been easy to assemble a staff of fine doctors, accredited specialists in eye, ear, nose, throat, skin diseases, orthopedic and other disciplines, all working without pay during the evenings throughout the year. I could not imagine what the Ethics Committee was charging us with which would prove so serious that it would drive more than half the staff to resign overnight. Compared with all the other difficulties I had experienced, and they were many, this was the most sickening.

When I talked to the doctors they all gave me the same reason for resigning. They feared the consequences of serving in an institution that could possibly be classified as unethical. However, after I recovered from the shock, twenty-four hours later I called and made an appointment to see Dr. Bowers, and I confronted him with the letter to Dr. William Wheeler. Dr. Bowers had one short answer, "The staff mis-understood the communication." *The entire staff?* He addition-ally stated he was merely seeking information concerning the administration of the Clinic and the functioning of the staff. I emphatically told him that the confusion was an intentional misrepresentation intended to convey to the majority of the staff that it should resign. I could not accept the letter as anything but injurious, intended to stop the Clinic from functioning. Dr Bowers relented.

There was never a week I did not have to face critics or representatives of ill-disposed institutions imputing the worst motivations to us. I knew my membership in the Medical Society was vital regarding my clinical work and in my association with the Clinic staff and other medical institutions. At all times I had to be on the alert regarding ethics in my own personal conduct, professional practice, and the operation of the Clinic.

One day, in 1932, for example, a committee of the Society summoned me because a Dr. Ott was giving training in physical therapy elsewhere and charging for his course. The committee took exception to free training at the Clinic for physicians. I pointed out that our notice was accepted and printed in the Massachusetts Medical Society's publication.

Another time I had to appear because a doctor for one reason or another personally visited members of the staff asking them to resign. At the same time, members of the staff received letters from the Department of Public Health signed by Dr. Gaylord Nelson. He asked the physicians about their connection to the Clinic and if they still served as staff members. This was the same misleading, ambiguous pattern of Dr. Bowers' communication sent in 1933. The intent of the letter was to alarm and demoralize the staff.

One doctor on the staff gave me a copy of his answer. On January 22, 1933, Dr. Abraham Myerson wrote:

> *I have been associated with the Reconstruction Clinic [the charter name of the Clinic at the time] for years. I am also familiar with the situation in Boston at the present time . . . [So] far as I know no institution . . . gives physiotherapy or allied treatments at night. I believe there to be a real need for this kind of service to the working community of Boston. I see no reason why the Reconstruction Clinic should not be made into a corporation giving this service.*

This letter was from a man who became a Professor of Psychiatry at Harvard Medical School and who practiced with Dr. Harry C. Solomon, who was also to become a Professor of Psychiatry at the same school and who was later Superintendent of the Massachusetts Mental Health Center. Ironically, I now serve as a trustee of the Center by appointments of Governors Furcolo and Volpe. So there were outstanding physicians who knew the Clinic's worth and who defended it and me.

There was also another communication from Dr. Bowers dated April 1, 1933:

> *...I regret to inform you that my letter to the [Public Health Commission] which has been construed as a quasi-endorsement of your organization is open to serious criticism because evidence has been submitted to me that the Reconstruction Clinic is still open to serious criticism. I shall write to Senator Myles of the Committee a letter that will remove the impression that anything that appeared in that letter which could be construed as endorsing the Reconstruction Clinic is withdrawn. You had no right to assume that anything I said or may say represents the Massachusetts Medical Society. The only persons who can speak for the Society are its duly constituted officers.*

My question was, *"Wasn't he an officer?"*

So there were times I became embittered, because of letters — such as that from Dr. Bowers — which were personally injurious. In addition, I received a call to appear before Dr. David Cheever, who was at that time the Chairman of Ethics and Discipline of the Massachusetts Medical Society. He was the Surgeon-in-Chief of the Peter Bent Brigham Hospital where he had his suite for private practice. I called on him there. After greeting him, I asked the purpose of his call. He said, "What are you trying to do?" He referred to the Clinic, of course. "Why the clinic? Who benefits from it?"

Patiently and at length I explained the purpose of the Clinic, described its organization, the staff, the people we served. He listened and merely said, "Dr. Cohen, I don't believe you!" I replied, "Sir, you have just called me a liar!"

Immediately, I realized I could no longer shake off the meaning of all the appearances before the Committee of Ethics and Discipline and the years of harassment and interference by the Society. All this time I had tried to ignore what they were doing to me and to the Clinic. I had been trying to concentrate on my work and to conform to whatever the Society and other institutions required. *But they did not want the Clinic as a member of the Society.* The Clinic was an embarrassment and a threat, by taking care of a group of patients whose needs had been — and would continue to be, by them — overlooked in favor of those among the more affluent.

I could not acquiesce. I confronted him: "You, by your statement, are accusing me of a lie. Therefore, under no circumstances should you think you are forcing *me* to disassociate myself from the Society that you represent. I wouldn't associate with you anywhere, anytime, or under any circumstances as man to man. The only thing that saves you from bodily harm is the fact that when I was brought up in a little town in Romania, the first fatherly teaching I remember was not to show disrespect to our elders. So the only action I can take is to sever myself from you or anything you represent. You might have expressed a doubt, but you have no right to say I lied."

Then and there I decided to resign from the Massachusetts Medical Society. That was an agonizing decision, but I was compelled to make it on the spot. There was no alternative. My conscience told me I was right.

The only reason my resignation did not seriously affect the Clinic or its operation or my relationship with the medical staff was that the Clinic's history and its struggle to establish itself was now public knowledge. But this became another operational handicap, another burden to carry, along with all the other obstacles.

I admit that never *within my hearing* was there detraction of the clinical work, though many expressed a conviction that the doctors on our staff were making large profits (caring for the non-affluent!). Some even expressed the belief that I, as Medical Director, was financially enriched by the Clinic, whereas all these years I had been forced to deprive my family of luxuries and too often the necessities of life by borrowing and mortgaging everything I owned, including furniture and home. I gave most of the income from my private practice to the operation of the Clinic. Imagine how rich I was getting!

Little did the opposition realize that the more it attacked the Clinic and me, the more determined it made me to continue. Nor would my conscience or my obligation as a physician permit me to abandon the work.

I called a meeting of the medical staff, imploring those who resigned to attend. I brought to their attention the fact we had been carrying the notices in the *Journal* regarding the Clinic for at least three years, that it was an approved, ethical notice, that we had not used any notice of a commercial nature. I then asked that they reconsider and return. All but one returned — this was Dr. Leroy R. G. Crandon, my devoted friend previously mentioned. He was Surgeon-in-Chief of the Boston City Hospital, and the pressure upon him from the medical community was just too intense. I could not blame him. He had already done all he could for the Clinic and for me. There were those, however, who did not waver. For example, one physician who needed his hospital affiliation for his private practice and therefore for his family support did not hesitate and continued to serve with us.

One should not think of these physicians as martyrs. They were doctors dedicated to their profession and the belief that there was community need for their services. They knew the patients could not afford the usual doctors' fees and that unskilled workers could not afford to lose a day's pay.

Thus, despite the objections of many of the medical community, social agencies, and those such as Dr. Cheever or Dr. Bowers, steadily the Clinic's work became more widely known and accepted. Industrial leaders spoke favorably about us, as did a number of members of the medical profession. By allying themselves with us, some of these citizens gave us strength and added conviction that it was a necessity to overcome grievous complications. Peculiarly, the adversaries defeated themselves, for they helped the growth of the Clinic. The Clinic survived no matter how forbidding the opposition.

The struggle my father was living through had an increasing impact on our home life. I must have begun to be at least somewhat affected by tension and by anger, as snatches of intelligence penetrated the serenity of my childhood. The home I remember was one to which my father came for dinner, made sure he was with his children, and after my bedtime, would disappear, apparently to go to the Clinic to work — and eventually, by the time I was 6 or 7, to stay there and sleep. What I did not realize was that my father needed something away from the Clinic where he could relax and rest, away from stress and conflict.

My maternal uncle Joseph, a pediatrician, lived with us in Cambridge for a while. He was probably 10 years older than my brother Manley. Often, he would spend his time playing pool with my brothers when he was home. The small pool table was upstairs, in a room next to Mrs. Gannon's, so I would hear the Clinic mentioned by my uncle Joseph and hear him telling Manley and Alfred about treating children there. And occasionally I would also hear my mother talk to him about it, saying things which are unremembered now.

The truth was, as my brothers later told me, my mother was not fond of the Clinic. She did not like what it had done to her life, keeping my father away from home and diminishing the money coming into the house. My mother felt the Clinic to be responsible for having much to do with our separation from my father. And I imagine that, as conflict increased, my father's need to find respite further increased that separation.

The year that I was ten, we lived without seeing my father very much at all. I had my appendix out — my pediatrician uncle took me to the hospital from where we were staying for the summer. Someone (probably Manley) knew where my father was and called him to come home. I did wonder afterwards why he hadn't come to get me.

— Richard S. Cohen

CHAPTER SIX: NEW FRIENDS, NEW HOMES

With the success of our clinical work, our nine-room suite ceased to be adequate. We had to seek larger quarters, get new and more equipment, provide funds for a larger paid staff of assistants. We could no longer afford to absorb deficits by what money I could personally supply. Our treasury was always in the red, given the nature of our service. In fact, I do not recall a day from those years when the treasury was in the black. However, we boldly planned to make the improvements, and I started to search for outside funding.

I called one industrial leader and was astounded to hear, after his acknowledgment of our good work, that Dr. Charles Wilinsky, my old neighbor and colleague in general practice, now Medical Director of the Beth Israel Hospital, had advised him not to contribute when the leader asked Dr. Wilinsky's advice. As Chief of the Health Department of the City of Boston, Dr. Wilinsky had — some time before this — come and inspected our facilities and practice at the request of Mayor James Michael Curley, following which, Dr. Wilinsky had sent me a letter praising our work and service to the community as a medical institution. When I telephoned Dr. Wilinsky to ask the reason for the turnabout, considering his letter of praise — which I read to him over the phone — he answered, "I told him to give it to *our* institution instead, and he did."

His betrayal did not stop me from asking others for financial help. I next went to the owner of the JA Cigar Company in the Huntington Avenue Building and asked him to contribute. Kindly, he informed me that although he knew we were doing good work and that our service was needed, he had been told not to give to the Clinic. I asked, "Who?

Why?" I could not help myself, considering that many of his employees came in the evening after working hours, thus preventing no loss of production to him. This was unquestionably a financial benefit for his company which should have made him well disposed toward the Clinic, my plan, and me. He said, "Doctor, I think maybe you *should* know." He telephoned Mr. Milton Kahn, Director of one of the large charitable fundraising organizations and told me he would allow me to listen in on the conversation. In a very loud and emphatic voice, Mr. Kahn, his personal friend, said, "Don't give them a nickel!"

Another example of what faced us in seeking financial support was my visit to the president of the Hood Rubber Company, a very major Massachusetts employer at that time. I took with me the case histories of about fifty employees of that company who had come to be treated at the Clinic after hours during that year. Calling in his medical officer, who conducted a small clinic offering limited services for employees, he listened to my explanation of the indispensable nature of the specialized aid in gynecology, eye, ear, nose, and throat, skin and other areas that the Clinic provided his employees. He told me his company was a large-sum contributor to the Community Chest and that he, like other industrial leaders, had been assured that all they needed to do was to give to the Community Chest, which served all recognized charities in the Commonwealth. However, the evidence I brought was impossible to ignore — that we received nothing! Stepping out of the office, he returned saying that officially he could not make such a gift, but, "Here is a cashier's check for $500." In such a manner he supported our work.

Here, then, was a new kind of post-graduate training in which I had to specialize — funding solicitor. To be sure, it would require more of my time and take from my other duties. I would also have to learn to be a star salesman. It was indeed a new experience. But who could tell the story better than I? Encouraged by some of the trustees, as well as by persons outside the Clinic family, I was beginning to be seen and heard where I could be most effective. Accordingly, I went to labor organizations. They held their meetings in the evening, and they understood my story. They knew they received benefit from the Clinic, that the Clinic helped them. They listened when I spoke at their annual convention and told me health was their *only* asset, that health should become a kitchen commodity, that it should be on the kitchen shelf above the breadbasket. They responded and helped.

There were others, many splendid members of our community: clergymen, industrialists, welfare authorities who befriended us, some joining our Board and Advisory Committees. Alice Stone Blackwell said of the Clinic, "I know it is doing admirable work which I believe nobody else in Boston is doing. I am very glad to do anything I can."

Mr. Harry Grages of the Boston Central Labor Union stated:

We regard your Clinic as doing indispensable work for the laboring people of our city. Large numbers of working men and women must attend a clinic after working hours. Yours is the only general evening clinic (part pay, part free) medical and surgical in Greater Boston. Many low-waged workers cannot afford the full cost of treatment, but their self-respect resents charity, and they want to pay the little they can afford. As you go to the public for support, you can count on the full cooperation of organized labor.

Among those to whom I most particularly express my thankfulness is William G. O'Hare, Secretary of the Public

Health Department, City of Boston. He joined our Board and said to me one day, "Keep trying. Keep working. You're doing grand work." I always remembered how he continued: "I've never seen a work that spelled out so strongly *the salvaging of human endeavor.*"

On another day, the Reverend George L. Paine, descendant of Robert Treat Paine, a signer of the Declaration of Independence, wrote, "A working man especially thanks this organization for being open evenings so that he does not have to lose a day's pay." And Bishop Wright said, "I sincerely meant the words of praise I spoke for you personally and for your associates in the wonderfully humane work you are doing. I wish you every blessing."

There was also Mr. Henry E. Hamel, who at this writing has served for more than twenty-five years and who is now president of the Board of Trustees. Throughout the years he always appeared in times of distress and depression. When he found me in despair, he asked prayers for me in church; and he always had words that were consoling, kind, cheering. It was as much as if he came to dress my wounds and doctor me.

Nor later could I forget the encouragement of his eminence Richard Cardinal Cushing, when the work seemed hopeless and I was discouraged. He put his arm about my shoulder and said, "Doctor, what would you think of me if I said I would like to quit?" Then, to punctuate his exhortation to carry on, he made the third contribution of many thousands of dollars, as he had done twice before. He also wrote congratulations and made a statement that removed doubt for all time about my ability to carry on. "I am delighted... because you have dedicated yourself to this great work. God be with you in all your way."

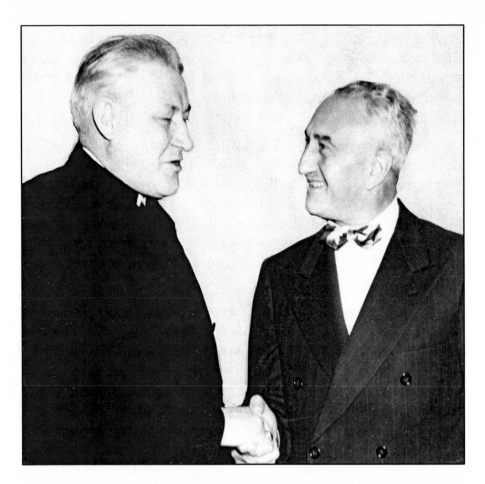

Cardinal Cushing with Morris A. Cohen

For some time now, we had been seeking a new home for the Clinic, one large enough for our expanded services, increased equipment, and additional staff. When we found the building at 452 Beacon Street, selling at the Depression price of ten thousand dollars, we faced the dilemma of not possessing a cash reserve for a down payment. One of our admitting clerks, Ms. Philadelphus, loaned the Clinic two hundred dollars which we used for a deposit. After paying a real estate agent an additional one thousand as a down payment, he then requested that we pay more in order to obtain a bank loan mortgage for the ten thousand. We paid, and later discovered that the agent had dishonestly kept that money as a bonus for himself. But we had secured our first building. The receipt of that deposit bears the date August 30, my birthday, in 1934.

The building needed extensive rewiring, and this was done by Mr. Morris Vigoda, a close friend who knew of the Clinic's financial problems. He did the required work not only on the existing wiring but installation for physical therapy, x-ray, and laboratory equipment. The Clinic could not repay him for many years. He still tells me our credit is bad, but he continues to service us when called.

After the purchase of the new building, I continued to serve without pay. Of course, it was always personally difficult. Moreover, my private medical practice — which I continued for income — began to lose in the competition for time. The Clinic demanded clinical, administrative, and financial attention. I believe my perseverance came, at least partially, from a boyhood experience. I wanted the fruit near the top of a tree. Climbing toward the uppermost branches, I slipped and tore a deep gash in my left leg, the scar of which I still bear. Despite the pain and the blood, I got the fruit. Experiences such as these mold our activities and determination in later life, or at least, indicate the will to succeed.

So we had our new building. But we also had to equip it for an increasing patient load. We purchased a new x-ray machine, added physical therapy equipment, and additional up-to-date laboratory equipment. A contributor, Mrs. Redpath, gave us two thousand dollars which we used as a deposit on the x-ray equipment. As other contributions came, we used these for the other machines and toward the expansion of the new facilities.

The opening day for the new building was May 12, 1935. Governor James Michael Curley delivered the dedicatory address standing before a bronze tablet affixed to the building and which read: *Dedicated by the founders for the purpose of conducting an evening clinic for the low-waged worker, who must receive treatment after working hours at low cost or free if necessary.*

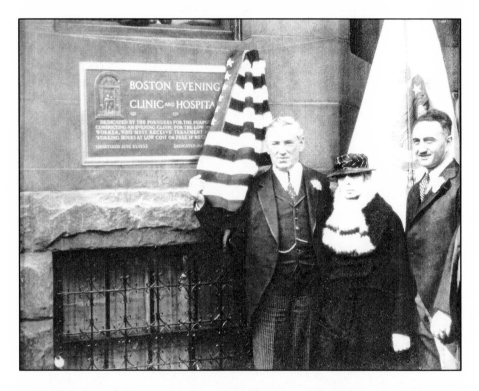

Dedication of the Boston Evening Clinic at 452 Beacon St., Boston, Massachusetts. From left to right: Governor James M. Curley, Alice Stone Blackwell, Morris A. Cohen

This milestone affirmed the validity of our new concept in health care and the work we had already accomplished and that which was to come. On August 29 of the same year, in a letter the Governor said:

It is pleasing to note that the Clinic is open to all people, irrespective of race, creed or color or residence, and that no patient is ever turned away because of inability to pay ... I am sure that the entire community appreciates the self-sacrifice of the unpaid staff of physicians, surgeons, and the members of the Board of Directors who are devoting their time and service for the benefit of the patients attending the Clinic.

Then, on November 25, 1935, we received a letter from the Minister Karl Heath Kopf of Mount Vernon Church:

I want you to have this word of gratitude from me in particular and from our Church in general for the gracious, cheerful and effective treatment which your Clinic has given to five persons whom we have sent to you within the last few months. To all of us it is a miracle that you can be so thorough and yet give your services so economically. I know of no other place where we can send the needy sick in the evening with assurance that they will be so kindly received....You must be under a heavy expense to administer your medical care at such low cost so that I hope you will get the financial support you so richly deserve.

Despite such praise, it was audacious to move to a larger facility because of the increased financial burdens, including needed repairs to the building. We were fortunate that our creditors were very patient and cooperative.

A recollection of 1936. There is a framed memento hanging in my office: on a small flag the text urges the re-election of "Franklin D. Roosevelt, Our next President," and over his picture it reads: "God Bless America." Below that is a photograph taken of his Packard touring sedan, top down, turning a corner. It was that same car that I saw, with the President in the rear seat waving and smiling to the crowds that lined Beacon Street. Before it drove past the Clinic, my father took my hand, walked me to the street, and made certain we would be standing at the curb as the President and his entourage drove by.

Obviously my father admired the President, but thinking back, I realize that he wanted me to see him. Whether I was thrilled or not is hard to remember, but I do recall the enthusiastic people and my father's smiling face as he held my hand. For me, it was the first and (to date) the last time I ever saw a President in person. Of course, our lives were filled with the magnitude of that man, his courage, and his belief in the people and their ability to withstand hardship and to stand by him. I believe that my father also possessed some of these same characteristics, and that it was determination and belief in himself that caused him to persist and endure in building and defending the Clinic. So that day, when FDR drove by with that typical smile and wave of his, he became a symbol to me over the years of what the Clinic and my father were: indomitable.

— Richard S. Cohen

Because of the finances, it was obvious that I would have to expand my effort regarding solicitations. There had to be professional appeals also. Moreover, I had to learn to become a convincing beggar. I believe now that the most disappointing, discouraging, depressing, and hardest part of my work involve-ed fundraising. It was burdensome, of course, considering my responsibility for supervision of all aspects of the Clinic's work. Nor did the detractors cease their harassment.

One evening, Mr. Basil Collins, Vice-President of The Old Colony Trust Company, a subsidiary of the First National Bank of Boston and a depository of the Community Chest, received a severe injury to one of his hands. Because he could not get to a doctor at that hour, someone told him he could go to the Evening Clinic to be treated, which he did. Because of this incident, he became interested in the concept of the Clinic. He occasionally chatted with me to learn more about the institution and our services to the community. I invited him to join the Board. He did. He was an active participant and eventually became Treasurer.

Sometime later I received a call from him telling me it was quite important we meet. When he came to the Clinic, he told me he did not know just how to begin but that it was necessary he tell me in person of an incident at the bank. His superior had told Mr. Collins that his service with the Clinic was a problem because of opposition in the community to our existence. Mr. Collins would have to make a choice: he would have to leave either the Clinic Board or his position as vice-president of the bank. With tears in his eyes, Mr. Collins told me how he felt, that leaving our Board was a most painful and regrettable action, but that he would have to resign and cease his activities at the Clinic.

Here, then, was one more instance of pain that was symptomatic of ignorant opposition to our patient services, *a symptom of an illness in the medical establishment and among members of the business community.* And all of this took place years after we received approval and the charter as a public charity. It made no difference; there were other citizens beyond reproach who not only helped the Clinic but also served on its Board. Yet it is unimaginable that citizens who could not benefit from services of the evening clinic because they could afford private pay would prevent or hinder medical help for the needy. Those in opposition neither tried nor made an attempt to observe and understand the services we performed. We were suspect for being too good to be true.

After this lamentable incident, all too reminiscent of Dr. Bowers' letter to the Better Business Bureau, we began to understand why it was so terribly difficult to get financial help. To this day I have never been able to understand or condone the behavior of people in positions of responsibility, those who demand our confidence, for turning upon or ignoring people in need who require, in our case, good medicine. It was this feeling of hopelessness regarding good deeds, aside from being called a liar, which also caused me to resign from the Massachusetts Medical Society. It was my obligation to review my purpose and to decide to exert more effort to assure the service we offered.

Admittance to the Clinic increased steadily. This was possible with additional space and personnel. It gratified us that in the publication of the Greater Boston Chamber of Commerce the writer praised the Clinic's good work and contribution to the business community because of our evening service: *"The Boston Evening Clinic saves thousands of man hours."* Yet, though the President of the Boston Greater Chamber of Commerce, Mr. Ernest Henderson, welcomed our *five hundred thousandth* admittance, the Chamber still advised businessmen to contribute only to the Community Fund!

To counteract such bias as exhibited by the Chamber, and to show that so many working people were benefiting from the Clinic's services, at one of our Board meetings Mr. Danforth suggested we should begin to place on the patient history card the name of the employer. This would give factual support of our health services to the particular industry. This made even more sense when one considers that patients came from more than two hundred communities outside the Greater Boston area and returned as healthier workers sitting at workbenches or standing at production lines. Yet, repeatedly, I had to tell employers that their workers — the elevator operators, bundle wrappers, stock clerks, janitors — did not receive ample wages to afford medical care, not even the low fee charged by the Clinic. They had to be treated free of charge. Therefore we required gifts from industrial employers. It was here that Mr. Danforth's suggestion proved valuable — so that we could convince the companies, particularly those in certain industries, that it was they who benefited most and that they should support us for their own economic benefit.

Confronted with such truths, as the President of Hood Company had been, they were beginning to accept their responsibility. But while the company executives may have begun to recognize the value of the Clinic, there was still a struggle regarding the Community Fund. A bit of history explains this part of the continuing conflict with this major fund gatherer. For example, the question most often asked of us in the 1930s was, "Why don't you join the Community Chest?" Of course the idea of a relationship had occurred to me, because there would be release from the strain of fundraising. I'd be able to stop begging. What a treat! — However, the prerequisite for membership in the Fund was membership in the Council of Social Agencies, the approval body. We filed the application for membership in the Council and met with the committee. Yet there was more. It was the unforgettable day I visited with Arthur J. Roche, Executive Secretary of the Council and Treasurer of the Permanent Charity Fund. The occasion etched itself in my mind. I talked and answered questions for at least 20 minutes regarding the Clinic and its administration. At no time did this man raise his eyes to look at or meet mine. That I was speaking honestly and of doing good for people and that he sat as he did, as a representative of approved agencies chartered for the same purpose as ours, was terribly distressing. Though this was one of the more melancholy moments of my career, afterwards I decided there was only pity for a man so unmindful of the presence of another human being.

My pity also extends to such people who spread or believed gossip about what was wrong with the Clinic, such as misappropriation of funds. This is and has been one of the worst lies about the Clinic and its administration. Moreover, charities listened to the medical organizations and banks that still talked against us. Those charities feared they would lose what they were receiving, at least as I see it. Thus, we did not receive acceptance at this time in the Permanent Charity Fund.

In later years, the Permanent Charity Fund did make contributions to the Clinic, but their earlier rejection gave many an excuse for not contributing to the Clinic. It was a problem trying to answer the repetitive question, "Why do you have to go begging for support for a service so needed and so beneficial to workers?" — Why indeed.

Perhaps one of the most traumatic experiences that children experience is the separation of their parents. What the problem was between my mother and father, before I was old enough to understand, I can only guess. However, later I could put together fragments of what my brothers told me, especially George and Manley at first, then Alfred. Of course, I had no idea what marriage was, only that my father was there when needed. He would leave the Clinic at any time if one of his children were ill. He was always there through my bouts with pneumonia and whooping cough, it seems. And on weekends, if he wasn't somewhere else, there were often picnics. He was, however, "somewhere else" more and more frequently. My mother and father had been separated for a number of years when Chloe came into his life. One weekend my father was going away, and George had to drive him to North Station. I went with them. As my father walked toward the station, I asked George, "Where is he going?" George answered "He's just taking the weekend off. He needs to rest," but he knew Dad was going to New Hampshire to see Chloe, our future stepmother.

His visits with Chloe were why we often had the car on weekends; and on a number of occasions, George drove my mother, sister, and me to New York to visit our maternal grandparents and Alfred, who was by now working in New York, beginning a career as an artist that gave him some later advertising fame. During these outings, there was never talk of divorce or of my father, only what we would be doing in New York, where it was always an adventure. However divorce had to have been in the background as far as George and my mother were concerned — for Alfred and my eldest brother Manley, as well. I doubt that my two older brothers ever said much to me, but I have the idea that my third oldest brother, George, knew much of what was happening and why. I see him in some ways as complicit, like Anna Roosevelt, FDR's daughter, arranging for his mistress to be in Georgia with him.

— Richard S. Cohen

CHAPTER SEVEN: WAR AND UPHEAVAL

In the early 1940's there were significant events that occurred to expand awareness of the Clinic. This eventually brought about a need for larger quarters, and while this was a concern, fortunately, such growth brought with it the desire of more good physicians to affiliate with our staff.

Then, one day in early 1940, our chief allergist and I visited Dr. Stratton about publishing the Clinic as a postgraduate institution, a title given to various medical institutions in the Greater Boston area. The Massachusetts Medical Society urged its members to participate. During the meeting Dr. Stratton raised the issue of my resignation from the Massachusetts Medical Society. A bit later members of the Society approached some Clinic staff and suggested my return.

When our medical staff met, they unanimously stated I should rejoin. As I recounted the reasons for my resignation, they said, "That's old stuff." My answer was, "I'll do so on the condition that the Society's records include a notation on how financially ruinous the Clinic had been to me personally."

Filed with the society, the statement included that I had founded the Clinic at the cost of personal anguish and funds to the extent of one hundred thousand dollars, and further, that my work resulted in neglect of my family interests and finances and my practice. The statement also included that in 1938, forced to give up my practice, I reluctantly, at the insistence of the trustees, accepted an annual salary of twenty-five hundred dollars as Medical Director. In 1941, the trustees raised that sum to thirty-five hundred dollars, and in 1943 to five thousand. With this information on the record, the Massachusetts Medical Society granted my readmission.

Yet, the personal cost continued to be great — to us all. My father had met another woman, one of the reasons for his frequent absences from the home. The woman who would replace my mother in his affections, Chloe, had fled Anatolia with her family when the Turks invaded. She attended Simmons, and was older than most of the seniors. (My mother also attended Simmons for at least a year and had left because of family responsibilities, a pattern repeated when she attended nursing school, before college. I believe that her time at Simmons must have made her even angrier about my father and Chloe.)

The earliest I heard the word divorce was not from any of my brothers but from my mother. There is no doubt that the Clinic and my father were irritating her and eating away at my mother's better nature. Sometimes she became just nasty, something I noticed later on. I realized then, not before, what was happening to her and how she must have felt as a woman whose husband cheated on her and who took another woman to be his partner.

One day my mother told me, "Your father wants to leave us, but I won't divorce him." I thought she was doing the right thing, at least at first. What I did not like was that her sister was her lawyer, but what did I know at 13 years old? I knew much about her sister. Aunt Jessica gave the impression of superiority, was involved in politics in the town in which she lived and thought of herself as outstanding and commanding. Her word was the word of God handed down from the mountain. And she said, "Don't give him the divorce. We'll take him for everything. My friend the judge will help." To this day I don't know on what bench this judge sat, but I had to meet with him; and when I did meet him, I despised him for the questions he asked, which were meant to damn my father.

"Did you ever see your father hit your mother?" "Did he ever throw her down?" NO! I have never forgotten my anger or dismay

or even how my sister, Selma, the youngest, and I reacted. It was as though our world exploded.

It wasn't until about the time of the divorce that I can remember my mother ever saying anything negative about the Clinic in my presence. On that day all I recall is, "That goddamn Clinic has been a curse, as has that other woman. I hate them both and him as well. I'm not going to suffer because of them." But she did – continually. And because of the shame and stigma of being divorced, she warned me never to say to anyone that she and my father were now legally apart. The effect upon me was difficult, for I knew it was a lie, and when friends' mothers asked me how things were at home, of course they were looking for gossip. I would tell them, "Everything is just fine." Of course, divorce then was a terrible disgrace for women, who were made to feel themselves unworthy. Society frowned on divorce. (But emotionally, those days are not any different from today with respect to women who have been blindsided by their wandering husbands or partners, except that the divorce rate has increased, and we read so much more about it.)

It was also obvious as I began to understand more that my mother was living a bitter life and did so until she moved with one of her sisters to Florida.

Of course, my father also had a responsibility to explain what was happening. Then one day I was alone with my father. Often he would take me to the Clinic, where he lived by himself. It might be during the week or on a weekend when he would take me to a movie alone or along with George, later Selma when she was old enough. On this particular day after he had seen some patients during the day, he called me into his office. At some point he said, "I've been asking your mother for a divorce. I've promised her everything she needs, including a house in Brookline." What he had chosen was a house on what was called, at least then, Summit Road or Hill, a beautiful house seen from the outside. But my aunt *still said, "No!" My mother, even though she was older and more experienced, listened — and said "No. Never." That was my mother's mistake — from which part of my bitterness arose, unrecognized until some years later, for we had been deprived of our usual pleasures, such as summers away, and a much nicer home.*

Anyhow, in my fourteenth year, he went to Reno and soon after married Chloe. Then my anger at my father intensified. He and Chloe rented an apartment in the Fenway. Perhaps those were some of the happiest days for him, to be free of the responsibilities of the Clinic and the fights it caused in the medical and social communities. But that made little difference to me at the time. I swore I would never see him again after they married.

But George, the advance guard, one evening asked me to go to the Clinic to see our father. I told George my father could go to Hell. George patiently explained that dad loved us and wanted to see me. He kept at me until I surrendered. George drove us to the Clinic. I dreaded entering, sat there among the patients until my father was free later in the evening. During that time, my anger rose. After a long while, George, who helped out in optometry at the Clinic (he was in optometry school at the time) came to me and told me Dad was waiting. I slowly walked to his office on the first floor, opened the door and stood there glaring at my smiling father. With no other thought but to tell my father I hated him, I stood in the doorway, looked at his smiling face, and told him "I don't ever want to see you again." Then I turned, holding the edge of the door, and slammed it shut. George then drove me home, criticizing me all the way.

But my father was an unusual man, and it took me time to realize just how much. He never surrendered. Shortly after that rude event — and it would never happen again, for I, too, was horrified by what I had done — my father called me and asked if I would come with him to the apartment for lunch on a Saturday. When we went in, I was fairly apprehensive and still cool to him. He asked me to sit in the living room while Chloe was getting lunch. I sat and waited. Soon, a tall, strikingly beautiful woman came into the living room and walked over to me as I was sitting on the edge of my chair. She talked to me softly, introducing herself, asking me questions about what I liked. Of course, the softening tactic worked, and in time, Chloe became a very important and loving person in my life. She led me to literature and, to an extent, away from the study of medicine.

What this illustrates is that my father, when determined — as he was with the Clinic — could accomplish what many others could not. It was a man like this who grew in stature and created a clinic that became so well known and who achieved so much in health care long before his time.

— Richard S. Cohen

The war years introduced new shortages, difficulties and uncertainties, personal as well as clinical. With pride and anxiety, one by one I sent three of my sons off to World War II to serve in the European Theater.

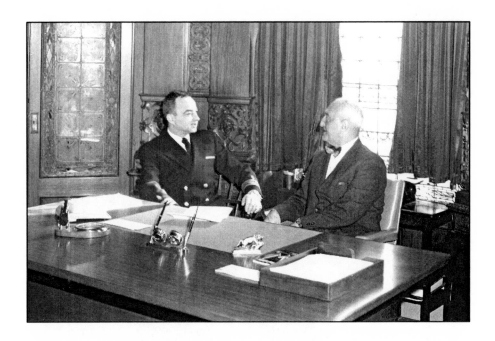

Morris A. Cohen with son George, who fought at Anzio aboard a minesweeper, YMS 16, was at Salerno and in North Africa and who retired a Commander from the naval reserve. Afterwards, he worked at the Clinic and then began his own practice in Cambridge, followed by his practice in Gloucester, Massachusetts for about forty years, retired and died there in 1997. He is pictured here in uniform on left, in Morris Cohen's clinic office, around 1950. George was then volunteering in the eye department of Chelsea Naval Hospital.

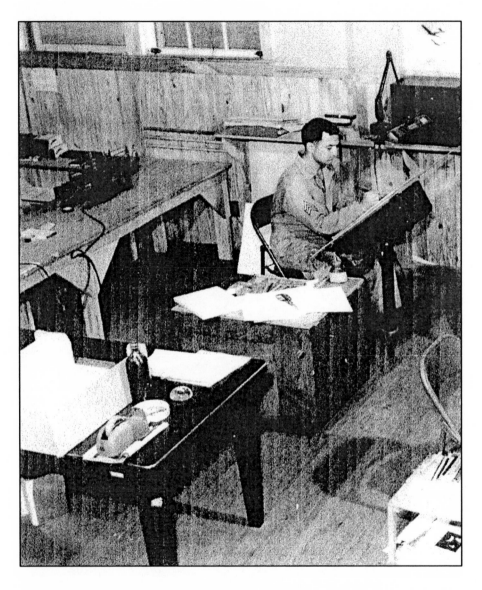

Alfred at drafting table in Moultrie, Ga., c. 1943, before going to England as a member of the Army Air Corps in WWII. Alfred was unkillable in a B-17 episode and buzz bomb attacks, was later recognized for his art and poetry and died in Amarillo, Texas in 2000.

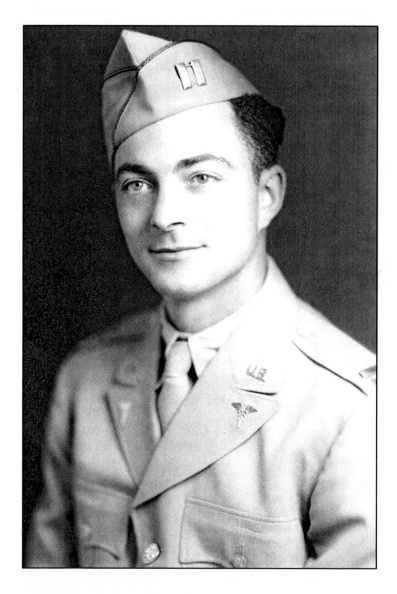

Manley Cohen, entering the Army. During World War II he later became a major in the United States Army Medical Corps, in which he won two purple hearts and a Bronze Star. Afterwards he continued with his training in thoracic surgery and practiced in El Paso, Texas.

I was fully reconciled with my father by the time I was seventeen and had begun working in the Clinic. When I walked in one afternoon after school, my father was giving a physical examination to a potential cab driver. He did this for a friend who owned The Checker Cab Company and probably was paid very little for the work. My remembrance of this exam was that he told the man he had too much fat and that he could hurt his back driving long hours. At least that is how I remember the conversation.

Soon after, when we were alone, my father said he had a job for me delivering x-rays to a court hearing. Apparently a patient was disputing the diagnosis of a doctor from a practice other than that of a physician at the Clinic.

"Dick, do you want to make five dollars?" Of course!

"Well, take my car and deliver these to the court. All you have to do is go in and hand them to the lawyer when he asks for them." Well, that was easy enough. The court was on Beacon Hill and not too far to drive, plus the money would give me something for a movie date and then a bit to save.

I found the courtroom and was told by a guard to take a seat and wait until I was called. That happened soon. I walked toward the lawyer and then was astonished to hear him say, "Please take the stand."

Someone said, "Raise your right arm." Then, "Do you solemnly swear . . ." This was a surprise. My father had not told me I would have to do anything but deliver the envelope with the plates. Once on the stand, the lawyer dramatically drew the plates from the envelope. "These are the x-rays of Mr..."

"I presume so. Those are the ones I was given."

"Now look at this," he responded and put one before my face.

"What do you see here?"

"I don't know. I was just told to deliver these." I was getting defensive.

"What disease do you see in this picture?" he insisted.

"I don't know. I'm not a doctor," I objected, but he kept at it. "Tell me!"

At that point I looked over at the judge. "Judge, I'm not a doctor! I was only asked to deliver these and that I would be paid five dollars. I can't answer his questions."

The judge started to smile. "You can step down and collect your money."

The judge gave an instruction to the lawyer who reached in his pocket, found a five-dollar bill, and gave it to me. I walked out of the courtroom, a little shaken but also smiling at the foolishness of the lawyer. You see, I had already had some experience with lawyers and judges before my mother and father's divorce, and based on that had nothing but contempt at the time for the legal profession.

When I got back to the Clinic, my father was still in his office. "Dad, you won't believe what happened to me in court," I told him.

My remembrance was a loud laugh and, "Did you get your money?"

— Richard S. Cohen

CHAPTER EIGHT: A NEW ERA BEGINS

In March 1948, one of Boston's most highly respected journalists, Rudolph Elie, after personally visiting the Clinic, wrote a feature article in *The Boston Herald* praising the Clinic. The following are his impressions as a first time visitor:

It's pretty wonderful when you think about it, how many things actually go on in a city that are really good and noble. We read in the papers most of the time of the bad and cynical things: we criticize, make sly suggestions that things aren't what they seem, pass on a bit of rumor or gossip and impute the meanest motives to everyone. Yet how do we account for such places as the Boston Evening Clinic... and all other numberless little charities, causes, institutions and philanthropies we see advertising for funds from time to time in the newspapers?... For all these do exist to a very large degree on man's humanity to man....

In a way, perhaps, the Boston Evening Clinic exemplifies the charitable institution that goes quietly about its way of offering medical assistance to those for whom the financial burden of private medicine is just a little too hard to bear. Thus, to its fine Beacon Street headquarters three (sometimes four) nights a week come hundreds of men and women. In the course of the clinic's 20 years, nearly 200,000 have benefited from its professional medical and surgical services.

Dr. Morris A. Cohen, Medical Director of the non-profit, privately endowed, publicly supported institution, told me, as we walked through the hospital-in-miniature that the patients pay 50 cents and no more for the services they require. "If that's a hardship," the physician explained, "they pay nothing at all. We have our own dispensary services for medicines, and we charge only the actual cost for the materials. But even there," he smiled, "if it means hardship, there is no charge. The clinic specializes," he continued, "in offering medical assistance to people who cannot afford to give up time from their jobs to attend daytime clinics."

All told, about 50 doctors serve on the staff, all eminent specialists in their field. The clinic also operates a training school for physical therapy technicians, and maintains a complete clinical laboratory... But most impressive to me, as I walked through the immaculate five-story building was the privacy, the air of poise, and dignity. "Well," said Dr. Cohen with a quiet smile, "medical science can do many wonderful things these days, but even medicine cannot cope with humiliation. Our first duty to our patients is to spare them that. Then we can only do our best."

This was the beginning of a new era for the Clinic in many respects. Admittance had increased from just over thirty-five hundred in the first year to just under twenty-four thousand for the year in 1948. Another signal of growth was to be found among our listings of Postgraduate Courses offered by institutions for additional physician training. We emphasized our Allergy Department among the listings, for we had one of the largest such facilities in greater Boston, not excluding the bigger hospitals. There was an increase in the size of nursing, clerical, and technical staff, which enlarged the financial burden. We had to begin nominally paying most of the staff. We also had to raise fees to two dollars a visit for those who could afford it.

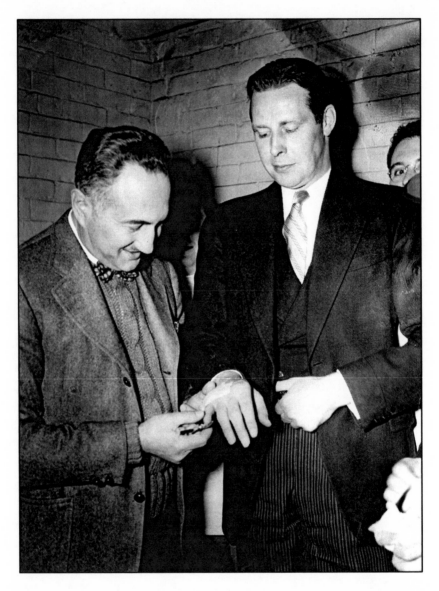

Morris A. Cohen is on the left, inspecting an apparent finger injury suffered by Governor Tobin, who served as Governor of Massachusetts from 1945 to 1947. Upon Truman's election as President, Tobin was appointed as U.S. Secretary of Labor, a position he held from 1948 to 1953.

Success and recognition of the Clinic also afforded much inner satisfaction. There is a story, so I am told, of a man who one night dressed in poor man's clothes and who spent some time in front of the Clinic stopping patients, telling them he was poor and needed medical attention, and asking did they think he could get good service, not being able to pay much. In this way he interviewed many patients entering and leaving our premises.

Being satisfied with what he heard, he had his accountant send us a donation of twenty-five dollars every month. His name was Irving Zieman, his occupation real estate. In 1950 when we found the new quarters we wanted at 397-399 Commonwealth Avenue, we discovered that Mr. Zieman was the owner. I visited with him and explained our pressing need for a larger building but that our deficit had continued to grow and that we had no cash. At the end of the talk, he said he would help us arrange a mortgage large enough to cover the purchase of the building.

A little later we found a purchaser for the Beacon Street building out of which sale we had a surplus of fifteen thousand dollars. Most of this we used for moving, necessary wiring, x-ray, laboratory, physical medicine, repair of the boiler, and other remodeling to change the new building into a clinical facility. The painters and plasterers union volunteered to paint the entire building, all its rooms and floors, or any other structural work. There were nearly fifty plasterers and painters assigned for the work that was done on weekends, both Saturdays and Sundays. All this took several years. The membership then gave us a party when they completed the work.

The budget for the building grew because of the size. Now, however, we found it somewhat easier to bring in funds. With the new quarters, the public image of the Clinic improved, as it did with the approval of supervising agencies of charitable institutions. There was also more public acceptance.

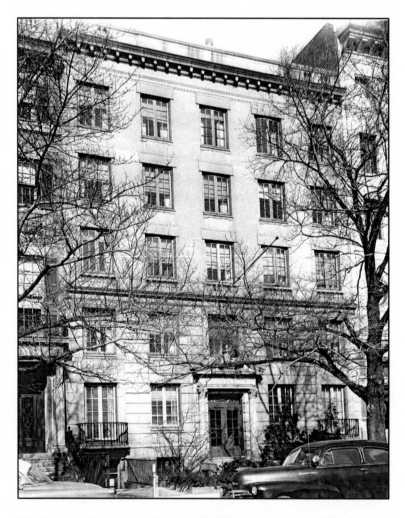

The Boston Evening Clinic, 397-399 Commonwealth Avenue

The health of the nation had become a national concern as early as the late 1930s, with the cost of health care passing ten million dollars. There was a movement for health insurance, but even as late as 1950, only fifteen percent of the cost of health care was covered by health insurance. By 1953, eight million families were in debt because of medical bills in the amount of one million dollars. Only one in every three families of those earning twenty-five hundred dollars per year had scanty coverage. At that time, only four percent of health coverage covered total medical costs. This meant that our work was even more significant.

In 1950, the National Research Council showed concern that sickness unrelated to industry was causing a loss of two million workers a year, the equivalent of more than five hundred million person days lost. At about the time of this report, the National Research Council issued another statement declaring, *"[P]reventive and timely ambulatory care in non-occupational illness is the only practical means for the prevention of absenteeism and disability from work"*

In view of all these statistics relating to worker and production effort, we, the Trustees of our institution, aimed to develop our resources to the utmost. Still, without any institution duplicating our work, such medical treatment nevertheless began weaving itself as a logical concept into the national health picture. Elsewhere, others began to see that our type of service had an invaluable nationwide application. Government and medical people began to visit us, causing us to recognize that we were engaged in something other than an isolated, regional venture in the practice of medicine.

We began receiving much more attention and the Clinic grew to a significant extent, also owing to the succession of patient allergy treatments for short intervals or for periods of months during a year. Because of us, the allergy patients in moderate- or low-wage income groups could stay on the job and receive evening care and remain symptom-free during work hours. In the various allergy seasons, a patient visited once a week for a period of months. Thus, before antihistamine drugs came into use, we had more than two hundred and fifty allergy patients in one evening. Our service was enormously valuable to mothers who could bring their children during the evening, after the fathers had returned from work and could stay home to supervise the other siblings. The attendance of this group was so great that we had to open a Children's Allergy Clinic.

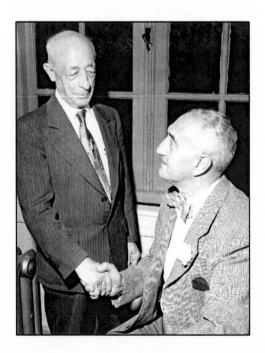

First Patient — The first patient (at left) admitted to the 397-399 Commonwealth Avenue Clinic shakes hands with the Medical Director, Morris A. Cohen.

Also listed in the Post Graduate schedule was our new Cancer Detection Center, started in the early 1950's. This was because we operated it under a group practice schedule – that is, surgeons performing the proctoscopies and sigmoidoscopies; physicians performing the medical examinations; gynecologists doing the gynecological examinations and pap smears. In such a way, examinations were carried out by specialists in each field, those more qualified by theory and practice than general practitioners in private practice. Thus, the pathology would more likely be detected.

We were also receiving larger contributions. For example, Mr. Alfred Avery contributed fifteen thousand dollars to establish the Cancer Detection Center. The Charles Hayden Foundation gave us a twenty-five thousand dollar grant for new equipment, including late model examining tables and updated laboratory instruments and microscopes. The award statement from the Hayden Foundation read: *"To be applied to your operating requirement and also the creation of new facilities described in your letter."* Gifts such as these gave us greater inspiration and confirmation of the validity of our purpose.

The new Cancer Detection Center was an outstanding addition to our services, making us also a prototype in the Boston area and beyond. It was the only such center in the geographical area – perhaps the *only* Cancer Detection Center not only in this community but probably within the state – that operated evenings. The multiple examinations we did comprised all necessary lab work, pap smears, chest x-rays or any further required x-rays, and took nearly two hours to complete. Statistics showed that seventy-eight percent of cancer could be cured when discovered early, whereas in the later stages only eighteen percent were curable. These percentages go along with the fact that in this department we examined asymptomatic patients only for diagnostic purposes.

The findings then went to the referring or family physician.

We performed these examinations at a charge of ten dollars (we now charge thirty-five dollars for such complete examinations, less for those unable to pay the full fee, or for free if necessary). Occasionally a member of the public would convey appreciation for our services in ways we could not have imagined, as expressed in the following letter:

Gentlemen,

Enclosed you will find a check for ten dollars. Each month for the balance of my life you shall receive a check for ten dollars on the 20th day. A few weeks ago I lost my mother after a short illness of six weeks. She was in the Carney Hospital for the entire period. While there she had nurses 'round the clock' and all the medicines and doctors that money could buy. After it was all over I thought what about the folks who could not afford this expensive care and treatment. "There must be a way." In a search, your fine service was discovered, therefore I wish to make this donation to you as stated above. May you be able to continue your service "Forever."

An article from this period titled "Healing After Dark," stated:

"Absenteeism because of illness alone," says the Boston Research Council of Economic Security, "[results] in the loss of service each year of 1 million workers and a production loss of two billion dollars." Furthermore, the Council report continued, "If all data were available, loss from absenteeism might be found to be as much as ten billion dollars ... Absenteeism due to illness is only part of the story, according to a statement by Dr. Robert G. Paige of New

York, President of the Industrial Medical Association. "For every employee absent because of illness, there are at least one dozen present who because of impaired health are merely going through the motions of doing something."

This last statement spells out in a very few words the situation which gave rise to the Boston Evening Clinic. Its schedule and low cost encouraged people to seek medical care rather than just going through the motions of their jobs in miserable working conditions. The report further stated that the Boston Evening Clinic, established 30 years previously "through the vision of its founder and present Medical Director, Dr. Morris A. Cohen, has labored increasingly to give timely care in every branch of ambulatory medicine and surgery."

A different kind of family memory – Morris Cohen, "the outdoorsman." In a move which also was to influence my own life profoundly, my father purchased a cottage (called a "camp") in Maine, on Embden Pond, a pristine lake surrounded by magnificent forests. He escaped there with Chloe, and frequently some or all of his children went with them. Attracted at night by the cottage lights, deer would come to the window, peer in, and rub their noses against the glass. Field mice would sneak in and stare while standing on their hind legs, their noses moving rapidly, then quickly disappear if you moved toward them.

We strolled down forest paths and met local residents who were different sorts of creatures than Bostonians. Among our neighbors were Fred and Irene Mullen, unusual people in our eyes, the kind you admire and wonder at, despite their having had no more than a high school education, if that. Fred was an expert mechanic who rebuilt wrecked cars. Once finished, you would never know the car had been in an accident. It was not just the shine and finish he gave the vehicle but an engine that ran as well as any new one.

Fred called my father "Doc" and rarely allowed anyone in his garage except a member of our family. Fred rarely talked and then in mumbles or half sentences, whereas Irene was far more voluble. They were exceptionally kind people, unaware of city social graces but with the goodness of human beings who care for others they deem worthwhile — kind, with rarely a harsh criticism of anyone, unless it was to make fun of someone who did something inane or extremely amusing in their eyes. Which, being city-bred people, I suppose we occasionally did, especially when we experienced country life in its more earthy form, such as, in the form of a hefty bear — like the one which sent Morris Cohen up a tree one day without hesitation.

— Richard S. Cohen

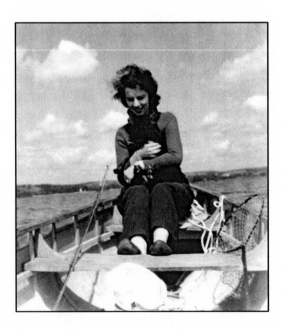

Chloe with poodle at Embden

While he, Chloe, and Fred taught us to treasure the quiet pastoral beauty of Maine, my father also taught us to fish. Fishing became, in fact, a prominent activity for all of us, especially Morris, whose reputation at it became legendary. He wrote a letter from the camp to George, who was in practice in Cambridge, Massachusetts, which said: "If you are coming up let me know when. I know you are busy and that's good. We are quite well here... Please go to Iver Johnson and get two (2) Brass No. 2 Dave Spinners — Those were one big spoon and two small ones, price $2.00 — I bought three before I came up here but that's all I have now — you can guess why — Really the kids [Selma and I] are having a great time... How are things at the Clinic?... We sure are giving away plenty of fish — Yesterday I fished with Soule while the kids were running around the lake in his boat found drowning at the head — when I brought Soule back lunch time — Mrs. Soule had cooked the two salmon I gave her as a surprise for lunch. I am taking the kids to Lakewood [then a well known summer play house] Wed eve..." (The play was "On Borrowed Time" with Thomas Mitchell, a wonderful actor.)

The outstanding value of this place to Morris was, no doubt, that it represented the apex of peace, harmony, and natural surroundings, affording him an opportunity to enjoy companionship and providing the perfect antidote to the stresses and pressures of his mission in life.

— Richard S. Cohen

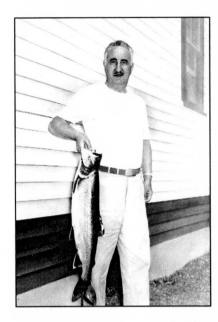

Morris A. Cohen, outside Sawyer's Market in North Anson, Maine, with his 14 pound largest Togue caught in Embden Pond to that date

Cottage on Embden Pond, in summer at right, in winter below

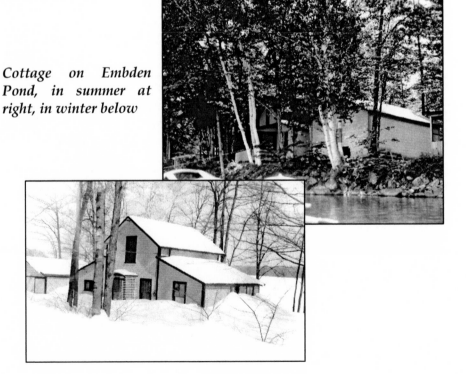

CHAPTER NINE:
STRUGGLE AND CANCER DETECTION

There was more recognition, as well as battles, to come.

On July 31, 1956, the Clinic gained institutional membership in the American Hospital Association.

We began receiving many more patients referred by other institutions, as well as from social service agencies – about twenty-seven to thirty thousand per year. The feeling of a new era of peace of mind from broadening acknowledgment by the medical and social service establishments was, at last, a modest but unreserved kind of gratification. But with or without approval, there was no difference in the conduct of the Clinic – we conducted medicine no differently than we had from the beginning and throughout the years since.

One day, soon after admittance to membership in the American Hospital Association, Mr. Myles, one of the directors of the United Community Services, made an appointment to see me at the Clinic. During the interview, he told me many civic leaders of the community, as well as representatives of institutions that were members of the Council, thought we should join the Council of Social Agencies and have a supporting membership in the United Fund. He said the Clinic would then not have to solicit independently to meet its deficit. The Clinic would then share in planning more economical and more effective community health programs. We would also be involved in *"the overall activities of the Health Division of the United Community Services which provides for the exchange of ideas and the opportunity for improving hospital and clinical administration."*

Further, he said, they accepted the Clinic as being

established as a completely outpatient, non-profit institution, that the Clinic had but one source of income — nominal, less-than-cost fee paid by patients, that hundreds of patients are accepted for less than the nominal fee, and that hundreds more received free care. He strongly urged we apply for membership in the United Community Service Council.

I hesitated, and reminded him that we had frequently been refused membership and that there was still opposition that made it difficult for the Clinic to carry on its work. The current opposition, I explained, was still prejudicial to the Clinic receiving support from the community. Further, because the Council was also recognized as an "approval agency," another entrance refusal would be a severe blow to the Clinic's ability to carry on. Therefore, I suggested to Mr. Myles and also to the Trustees, that we advise the Council that they act on the admission of the Clinic to the Council without an application. If the Council would then admit the Clinic, we would under this condition submit an application, if necessary. He left, saying he would try.

He carried the message well, for on July 2, 1957, they asked us to submit an application for their files. That letter was historic. We felt the letter highly significant in establishing the Clinic as a community medical and social service agency in the Greater Boston area.

We had two meetings at the Council offices preliminary to sharing in the distribution of Council funds to member agencies through the United Funds appeals. We submitted our budget, which stated the minimum amount of money with which we could operate, and a description of our programs. The Council sent a medical committee to observe Clinic operations and recommended approval of our procedures.

But at the final meeting of the Committee, they advised us

that because of the number of agencies to which limited funds were allocated in a rigid formula, the agency could only provide a small part of the Clinic's minimum requirement — about fifteen thousand dollars. This was a blow, because even without a fundraising drive of our own, we would still have a yearly deficit of sixty thousand dollars.

We told them we could not accept their fifteen thousand, as it would prevent us from soliciting supplementary funds, which in turn would limit our work and force us to stop offering the unduplicated services which they described as indispensable to the community.

In response, the Committee of the Council asked that we continue our membership as a non-financial member. There were one hundred and six other institutions in this category, of which twenty-five were hospitals but which held membership in the United Community Services as non-financial members.

Non-financial membership in organizations such as the American Hospital Association, Hospital Council of Greater Boston, United Community Services could help us to improve our staff with the finest physicians and surgeons. This would lead to growth and acceptance of our specialty departments because of a larger patient load. We accepted this course, and as a result, we soon needed to seek larger quarters again.

One justification for this move was that we believed the people should know of the existence of our recently-inaugurated Diagnostic Center, because it was a public health facility. With that in mind we met with Dr. John Conlin, then Director of the Public Relations Department of the Massachusetts Medical Society. We asked whether it was within the ethics of the Society to publicize the Cancer Detection Center. Because it was a center for diagnostic purposes only, not for treatment, he told us we could publicize it in the press or anywhere else we wished.

He did, however, give us an example from his own experience: when he received a federal grant for free diagnostic health examinations for purposes of prevention, he publicized in the press, in order to attract people supposedly in good health and unaware of any symptoms, but it was to no avail — the ads failed to persuade many people to come for diagnostic evaluation. Finally, he sent sound trucks through the streets inviting people to come to The Boston Dispensary to take advantage of the grant.

I tell this story as a preliminary to the later episodes in our cancer detection program when the medical society changed its mind in relation to our role. For, just about this time, the Department of Public Health began a fact-finding research survey to determine whether the State should establish and support cancer detection centers. We had already made application to the State to help finance the enormous cost of operating our department. Each examination that included doctors, nurses, other aides, x-rays, and laboratory work cost us twenty-seven dollars to perform, but we charged ten.

Not long after our application, the State announced its findings in an article in the *New England Journal of Medicine.* The conclusion stated that the State could not afford to support such clinics because the cost was too great. Soon after, the State Department of Public Health and Cancer Society advised that every doctor's office should serve as a cancer detection facility. This conclusion was, to us, and I would think to many physicians, completely out of line in such an important aspect of public health. How could a physician be expected, first, to give the required amount of time? How would he/she afford the necessary facilities for such examination, including x-ray and laboratory? Finally, how many would be qualified to perform such quality diagnostic procedures, such as we provided at the Clinic? From my standpoint, the State's conclusion was insensitive and unrealistic.

This was our contention for State support in our appeal to the Cancer Society. However, everywhere we applied we were turned down. This could not stop our work, however. Not only that, we eventually went from operating the cancer service from once a month to once a week because of the increasing numbers coming in and on the waiting lists. Many of our staff physicians went without pay, being content merely to serve. Many donated their compensation as a gift to the Clinic to help during our financial difficulties with the Cancer Center, as well as with our other services. I cannot recall one doctor discontinuing or reducing any service time because of the frequent financial problems. I myself went without salary for months at a time. We just continued what was important to us — providing health care without sacrificing quality.

Aside from the issue of our providing cancer detection, there was a continuation of opposition to other aspects of our work, opposition with which we were already quite familiar. There were always those who spoke ill of the Clinic. One experience seemed particularly devastating. One day I was called to the office of the Director of Hospital Facilities, a part of the Department of Public Health, and was commanded to stop using our Cancer Prevention and Detection Center. I pointed out that throughout the entire country there were such centers. In reply, the individual told me that the Clinic was not large enough to claim such a center. He would refuse to grant us the license to operate the Clinic that year if we did not adhere to his ruling.

With financial difficulties and other outside obstructions, we could manage to operate — however with this kind of intrusive threat, unprecedented after over twenty years of operation, there was no contending.

Silently I told myself, "I dare him to do so!" Well I could object in my mind, but I had to acquiesce to his demand.

We did receive our license — but six months later than customary. So, since the yearly license states we may operate until the next yearly license granting, I suppose we really operated the Clinic outside the law during the previous half year. Regrettably, that was not the only time there was a delay in our yearly license when someone thought we needed a rap on the knuckles.

Our experience stands as another chapter in the saga of the struggle for meaningful health care in this country, along with the opposition of the American Medical Association to President Johnson's Medicare program. Other major institutions and the Congress have not yet fully faced the reality of care for the needy, for the low-income workforce and aged citizenry.

But with continued adversity also came belated recognition. A revitalizing experience occurred: I was given a testimonial dinner, the chief speaker being the Lord Mayor Briscoe of Dublin, Ireland. Other speakers included Mayor Collins of Boston; Dr Lawrence R. Dame, President of the Massachusetts Medical Society; Dr. Alfred Frechette, Director of the Commission of the State Department of Public Health; and other eminent civic-minded leaders of Greater Boston. This is the letter Dr. Dame wrote to me on September 10, 1959:

Dear Doctor Cohen:

Physicians are most fortunate, in that they may daily have the opportunity to assist those who are in distress; in that their assistance is really desired by the recipient; in that they are received in an attitude of trust and hopeful co-operation.

When the period of acute personal suffering and concern has been alleviated successfully the patient and the physician have a lasting bond of mutual satisfaction resulting from this success. The longer a physician is to practice the more help he can give those who call upon him for help and the happier he is for his ever increasing skills.

To some physicians are given a special opportunity to demonstrate the profession's desire for greater distribution and improved care of the sick. History proves that in the field of personal ministrations one ever strives to justify the trust placed in him.

You have been one of those with a special opportunity and I am sure that you are glad that you persevered.

I am happy to join with others on this special occasion when your efforts on behalf of the sick are being recognized, and I trust that an additional glow will warm your life.

Sincerely yours,

Lawrence R. Dame, M.D.,
President, Massachusetts Medical Society

While the greatest compensation was the work itself, testimonials such as these lifted our spirits, validated our purpose and sacrifice, and encouraged us to keep going.

And there were other pleasant events, as well. One such occasion was a surprise party on the radio show *"This is Your*

Life." One of those presented to me appeared with his young wife. He asked, "Do you remember my father who came to the Clinic six years ago? Do you remember the small cancerous mass found in the upper lobe of his left lung and how Dr. Irving Madoff removed it?" He told me the family was overjoyed his father was still alive and carrying on a normal life. Who would ever think of giving up such work? I never did.

CHAPTER TEN:
PSYCHIATRIC SERVICE ON A SINKING SHIP

One very significant health factor we sought to address early on was the life of our citizens under economic imbalances that demand attention. Such imbalance causes great stress that affects productivity among millions of our citizens. The results are anxiety, depression, confusion, and frustration.

Eugene B. Gallagher, Ph.D. and Stanley Kanter, M.D. of our Psychiatric Clinic have done research, "The Duration of Out-Patient Psychotherapy," published in the *Psychiatric Quarterly Supplement*, v. 35, 1961. The problem they studied is common to many psychiatric clinics and is universally ignored, which is that the majority of patients become early dropouts. Doctors Gallagher's and Kanter's views are that the factor of early patient dropout is as significant as the treatment itself. Their findings in a comparison of four clinics were that the dropout rate in all was highest among patients of lower social status. There is great significance in this finding regarding the education that still must be accomplished before the non-affluent part of our society appreciates the advantages of modern preventive medicine.

The study also indicates to me the great significance related to the basis on which I founded the Boston Evening Clinic, as well as recollection in my earlier life that such a clinic would contribute to maintaining workers on the job. They had to be taught about preventive medicine, including the belief that there was a center such as the Clinic where they could be treated for a variety of health problems.

These doctors found that in comparison with the Veterans'

Administration Clinics, one in Baltimore and one in New Haven, the Boston Evening Clinic showed a *"relative decline in the propensity to drop out the longer a patient continues."*

Further, there is an alarming picture that shows that *"thirty-five percent of patients admitted to hospitals for psychiatric care would not become inpatients if given early and timely ambulatory care."* Of interest, then, is that our psychiatric department was the only one in the state providing evening ambulatory psychiatric care. Keep in mind also that most psychiatric patients require such care given frequently over a long period of time — months, sometimes years. Patients who needed the services of our clinic certainly could not afford to receive such care once or twice a week from private psychiatrists or psychologists. These patients are working under such stress and confusion that they could earn barely enough for necessities. They have come to us paying two dollars, one dollar, fifty cents, or nothing. Where else in the world could they go and receive such excellent psychiatric care for such a fee, and in the evening, to enable them to keep their jobs? The Clinic made this possible. They came in large numbers, and at larger cost for us because of the resulting need for psychiatrists, psychologists, and psychiatric social workers. Perhaps readers will be astounded to learn we had more than ninety such patients coming during one evening! It would become a civic tragedy if this unit were forced to close.

We could provide this service only through our Research Department, with a grant from the National Institute of Health, which we obtained, and which continued for four years. When that research project stopped, we discovered how costly that department would be to operate under the most ideal conditions, let alone one which never operated without financial stress: the deficit of operating just that one department was over twenty-two thousand dollars. It was inconceivable for us to sustain such a loss in just one department among the twenty units operating as part of the Clinic. On the other hand, how could we bear to see the tragic consequences of stopping, if we were unable to keep the department going?

It did become somewhat easier for me to obtain psychiatric personnel because of my appointment by Governor Foster Furcolo as a Trustee of the Massachusetts Mental Health Center, a teaching facility for the psychiatric department of Harvard Medical School.

At this time we were also in the greatest financial stress because we were always adding new services while maintaining all established services. And we never skimped on any service while adding another. Because of this, we found ourselves, in this particular year, with an accumulated debt of sixty thousand dollars, counting past years. Every creditor was quite good to us, saying, "We know the good you do, and that you will pay whenever you can." They all donated, in part, I believe, because they knew that it was the patients whom they were helping.

Troubles do have a way of snowballing, however. We found ourselves in a building that was sinking. Like so many hundreds of others in the Back Bay of Boston, the building was on landfill which had been added to part of the bay. The inspectors who came when we found that we could not open or close the doors stated that the structure was, as I said, sinking. We would have to close the building unless we took immediate steps to bolster the supporting beams.

Now wouldn't one say that this would have been a good time to quit? This would have been an excellent excuse. We didn't stop, of course.

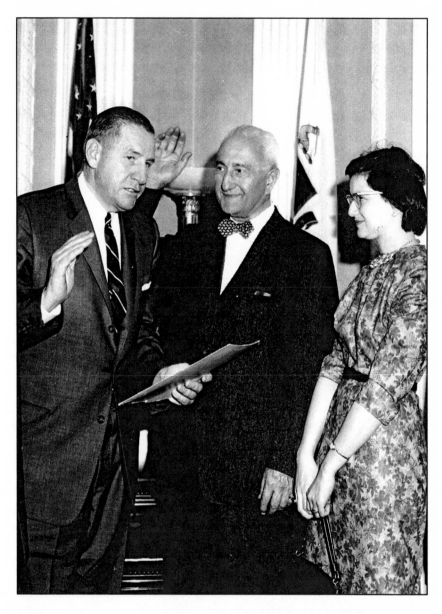

Morris A. Cohen being sworn in as Trustee of the Massachusetts Health Center, of which he later became Chairman. From left: Governor Furcolo, Morris A. Cohen, and his daughter Selma Cohen Goldfarb

Fortunately, an insurance company located next door needed space. They bought the building and put an emergency crew to work repairing it. Meanwhile, given permission, we continued to operate for a little more than a year on the premises, all through the structural changes — even when the buttressing required Charles River water to be pumped in twenty-four hours a day.

Once again, at this most critical moment financially, we were given the substantial help of a fifty thousand dollar contribution from Mrs. Laura McKinley Stackpole. A long time resident in the Back Bay, she became an early contributor through her friendship with Alice Stone Blackwell. The Trustees decided that this was our chance to redeem the faith which our creditors placed in us. We were able to pay off nearly our entire accumulated debt, and for almost the first time in one quarter of a century we were practically debt-free. We even had nearly ten thousand in cash left over, because of delayed discounts from those bills that had been paid. The debtors gave us this as a charitable contribution from the profits that they would have made had we paid in full. They charged us no interest but gave us a substantial reduction on the bills, thus saving us nearly fifteen thousand dollars.

There was an offset to the savings, in the great increase in size of our operating budget, which had grown to one hundred and twenty-five thousand dollars per year, with the patients still paying less than half of the operating cost — and somehow we never succeeded in our efforts to raise sufficient funds from contributions to meet our ever-increasing operational debts.

We had one pressing problem at this time. Where could we expand from here? Our workload was ever-increasing, our staff also. We now operated with nearly ninety people on our payroll. I was receiving ten thousand a year salary, for it was quite a few years since I had given up my private practice to devote all my time to the Clinic. We were also overstaying our welcome in the building that we sold. Obviously we continued looking for a new building. Finally, in 1959, we found an outstanding building for our needs only two blocks away at 314 Commonwealth Avenue at the corner of Hereford Street.

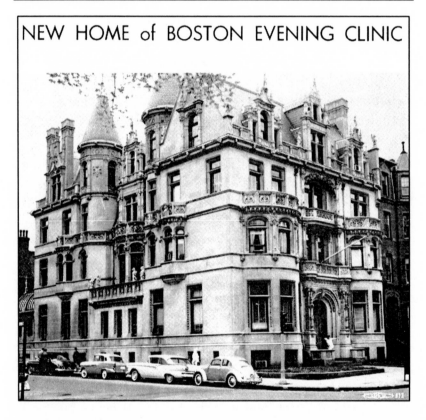

NEW HOME of BOSTON EVENING CLINIC

The new Clinic location at 314 Commonwealth Avenue. This building, called Burrage House, was — and is today — one of the most beautiful examples of architecture in the city. Numerous books have been written about it, and it has been featured on Boston walking-tours for decades.

Upon inquiry about the new building, the real estate agent told me they already had two deposits for the sale. This building seemed so suitable; I could not give up because of the information about the deposits, as there was little real estate in the area that could have housed us adequately.

I called the Phoenix Insurance Company, owners, at their office in Hartford, Connecticut and asked for an appointment to see Mr. Phinney, the head of the Real Estate Department. When we met I told him I was aware of the deposits, but that our work and our needs required such a building in that area. Further I made it clear we were under obligation to vacate our present building and had no place to go. I also told him of the great contribution it would be to our work, if they would help us obtain 314 as the new home for the Clinic.

In view of what I had told him, plus the endorsement letters from citizens known locally and nationally which I had shown him, Mr. Phinney said he would like to discuss it with the president of the company. He asked me to wait in his office, because the president was at that moment having a meeting with some of their executives. In about half an hour he returned to his office and said, *"Dr. Cohen, we have called a few people in Boston to inquire about the Clinic. We had such good reports of your work that we feel practically obligated to make sure that you can purchase the building."* He said we would need to pay down twenty thousand dollars toward the purchase price of a hundred thousand, the remainder being the mortgage which they would hold. With that agreement, I gave Mr. Phinney a check for one thousand. He accepted that. However, you may be shocked, we did not have that amount in the bank. So I started running around begging, and one man answering my plea giving nearly six thousand.

After that and within a month, just a few days before the

completion of the purchase agreement, I called Mr. Phinney and told him I needed to see him again. I now asked if there was some way they could accept only ten thousand as the initial payment and give us a mortgage of ninety. It was evident during the conversation that he knew quite a bit about the Institution and its operation. I also believe he had made it his business to find out quite a bit about me. Again, I waited in his office. On his return, he said that after talking it over with some of the executives in his department, they decided to accept. That was another happy day.

We now owned and were ready to occupy our new quarters. In our anxiety under the pressure to vacate the other building, we did not stop to investigate the problem of getting this building ready for occupancy. When we did, we found that laying of linoleum floors, painting, and some structural renovations amounted to more than ten thousand dollars. To repair the heating system and zone it more properly for our use required another twelve thousand. There was extra wiring and electrical work necessary in the amount of eight, and repair of the elevator would cost approximately three. Other minor repairs and moving would amount to over five thousand. We were now faced with a capital expenditure on the building of close to forty thousand.

But as you have seen in the past when emergencies arose, some severe enough to panic most, our faith in our work helped us to accomplish what needed to be done. At this time we received a gift, a non-restricted contribution of twelve thousand dollars from a former patient who had been a postal worker in the Cambridge Post Office. With this, plus a little more strenuous begging, we were able to make the needed repairs and have the building ready for occupancy; we moved into it in November, 1959.

New and added facilities always greatly increased our patient attendance. In turn that continually increased the deficit of our annual operating budget. So again, operating in the red, we started to prepare for operation in new quarters.

Some may wonder why we did not try to solve the deficit by raising the fees. It is because the Clinic had become known as a haven for those who could pay only part of the cost or nothing. The Clinic's purpose was to serve evenings, to prevent the added financial trauma of loss of a day's pay. We were militant about never humiliating the Clinic patients, about preserving their pride. By experience we found these people faithful to their obligations and sincere in their desire to pay what they could.

As an example, a woman from Cambridge, Massachusetts wrote, just before Christmas of that year, a letter which I quote exactly as written:

Dear Dr. Cohen,
Your letter was recently received and I know you are very good work. My dear friend, Dr. Evelyn Mitchell, one of the cofounders was dedicated to the work.

My brother and several cousins were in the medical profession all passed on so I know the need for your Center. I am a lone, elderly lady who has no income but a small pension. I've struggled alone to maintain myself in the family home — alone for 18 yrs. Had two House breaks the <u>last</u> shocked my already shattered nervous system and <u>conditions</u> over which I had no control forced me out of my home at an unfortunate time or might not have survived. I've been ill the last three months in the wk. Bout with severe case of intestinal virus that has left me so weak as I have little on which to build. The past seven mos. have been very difficult, breaking up, moving and getting adjusted small quarters in a new era just *about finished me along with wrenched and sprained ankle that did not help my already worn out physical body.*

It has and is a tough battle to restore myself to some what better state of health but with God's grace I pray that I may make it. I'm enclosing a small check to help in your work. May the Christmas season bring more hope to those in the sick world and I pray that the winter will be mild to help out in this energy crisis.

I am glad that you and the staff can continue your work. I would like to come for examination at some future time but it no longer is safe to go out after dark because of the increasing crime that has ruined our way of life.

May God's blessings be with you all and your institution always.

Sincerely yours, (etc)

Enclosed: Check No 222 on First National Bank of Boston for fifteen dollars

---

One of the most striking aspects of the Clinic's approach has always been its belief in a humanitarian response to the patient's inability to pay. I have been told by people that they never saw so many happy sick persons in any one place as at the Clinic. Such an atmosphere was created by the behavior of the staff — the doctors, nurses, technicians, all. It was often possible that a patient may have paid five dollars on admittance, but that money was all he had left. I have also seen a patient who was asked to pay something toward an x-ray and who replied, "I can pay only two dollars." This same young woman was then asked, "Have you got car fare left?" The patient had only thirty-five cents left in her pocket. Should we have continued to question this person and embarrass her further? Does not such treatment lead to uneasiness and frustration of the healing process? Should we have changed our policy? Others had; we did not.

To help us at this time in adjusting to increased operational costs, we had to entreat the capitalized Phoenix Mutual Insurance Company to let us suspend principal and interest payments for a six-month period. The company agreed to our request after appraisal of our circumstances. We had to place a second mortgage on the building. Worse still, we now learned that through some mistake, we were not included in the budget requirements in the Departmental of Mental Health. If we did not continue to receive financial aid from the state, we would have to close the department. We were advised to see the State Budget Director, who told us that if the Commissioner of Mental Health, Dr. Harry Solomon, would approve, a bill for special legislation could still be put through the Legislature as a supplementary budget for the operation of the Psychiatric Department of the Clinic.

When the Budget Director called in the Director of the Department of Hygiene, he expressed his regret that through an oversight we were not included and that he would be in favor of such legislation being put through in this term. However, Dr. Solomon was in Philadelphia delivering a paper. With only a few days left in the legislative session, legislators were approached, especially members of the Ways and Means Committee, who were told of the Clinic's dilemma and of its indispensability to the community as the only evening low-cost psychiatric clinic. The Legislature prepared a bill that Dr. Solomon approved upon his return. Voted on within a matter of days, this emergency legislation enabled us to continue. The state support went for salaries to psychiatrists, psychologists, and social service workers. The obligation of the Clinic resulting from the legislation was an arrangement for a full floor, five-suite facility, including salaries for its secretary and other help, for services, supplies, and utilities.

When the state enforced a new law we were not certain of recognition in its Mental Health Program, even though we were the *only* evening psychiatric ambulatory service in the community. Happily, we were included in the new set-up. In fact, there were recent expressions from the Mental Health Center that they wished to help our program. We received official confirmation that our chief psychiatrist, Dr. Alvin Stander, would be put on full-time pay so that he would have ample time to give his undivided efforts to an enlarged facility. With this recognition had come at last what I urged for decades in the concept of healing after dark — it was at last catching on and becoming a nationally recognized innovation in medical service. Hopefully, this recognition will create its counterparts in many states of our country. Aside from this, throughout the years, good days meant nothing more or less than the assurance that we could continue to operate our institution and make our unique contribution.

Although recognition in papers like *The New York Times* did not occur until 1965, an editorial by Harold Banks in *The Boston Sunday Advertiser,* January 31, 1960, stated that the work of the Clinic's effects are no mystery to Bostonians:

Honors have accrued to [Dr. Cohen]. He has been cited again and again by a number of civic, labor, and fraternal organizations. He has seen his beloved clinic accredited by the American Hospital Association and the Hospital Council of Metropolitan Boston, recognized by the Massachusetts Public Health Department, the American College of Allergy and the Post-Graduate Institute of the Massachusetts Medical Society.

Aside from advocating care for all, including preventive measures, I am happy to say that cancelling a part of the name of our Cancer Detection facility, and threat of cancellation of our license, did not stop our work. In fact our example of preaching and practice in the interests of the low-wage earner had also been supported by President Kennedy, who had been on an advisory board of the Clinic.

In an editorial headed "The Boston Evening Clinic," *The Boston Globe* stated on April 27, 1961:

President Kennedy, in one of his major addresses spoke with great urgency of the nation's immediate need for a vast network of community night-time medical centers for working people...

Perhaps it is no accident that a president from Massachusetts should bring into dramatic focus the great need for an after dark public health program which — for the past 35 years — has been pioneered by the BOSTON EVENING CLINIC.

For three and one-half decades the Boston Evening Clinic has provided desperately needed after-working hours medical care for over 800,000 men and women to whom loss of a day's pay in seeking treatment is as frightening as the illness itself. Every one of the 800,000 patients taking care at the clinic's 27 medical departments and Cancer, Psychiatric, and the Allergy centers have been treated at less than cost fees or at no cost at all. Amazingly enough there are many thousands of Bostonians who are completely unaware of this dramatic program of "healing after dark" functioning five evenings a week for their neighbors in 100 Greater Boston communities.

Perhaps it is because for these past 35 years the Boston Evening Clinic has been too absorbed in its quiet fight against great financial odds...

This medical center has sought to keep the lights of "healing after dark" burning solely as a beacon for the ailing and the depressed... NOT as a spotlight upon its achievements and its silent struggle to sustain and expand these achievements.

This month the Boston Evening Clinic celebrates its 35th Anniversary as the foremost full-time evening Clinic in the United States.

President Kennedy's urgent message places the Boston Evening Clinic in the spotlight it has long deserved. It would be fitting if the Greater Boston community should determine that the 35th Anniversary milestone of this haven of mercy and healing should also be the beginning of a new frontier of generous community support.

I was also presented by my good friend, the publisher of *The Jewish Advocate* and a Trustee of the Clinic, a copy of an editorial, "Evening Clinic's Anniversary," April 18, 1961:

In this era of the Organization Man to whom the single courageous act for an untested ideal or idea is not only outlandish but outmoded, it's exciting to see and give recognition to that rare individualist who is willing to go it alone for something he believes in.

Such an individual is Dr. Morris A. Cohen, founder, medical director and guiding spirit of the Boston Evening Clinic which this week launches its 35th anniversary celebration of "healing after dark."

The idea of after dark medical centers is now finding wide acceptance. But for three and one-half decades, Dr. Cohen, with obstinacy and perseverance, pioneered this vital concept.

Today the Boston Evening Clinic is among the foremost full-time evening clinics in the United States, offering a complete range of medical and surgical care, five evenings a week, at fees less than cost and, often for no fee at all, for hundreds of thousands of working people and their families in Greater Boston.

Through the efforts of Dr. Cohen, the light of "healing after dark" has been kept burning as a constant beacon for the ailing and depressed. One can only hope that the mold of a single man forged from the fires of an era when both poverty and a passion for one's fellow man were equally in vogue, will continue to inspire others toward idealistic ventures.

Financial woes continued unabated. At Christmas 1963, we had again to appeal to the staff to make contributions of their salaries for the month of December. Some of the paramedical personnel, nurses, laboratory technicians, physical therapy technicians, and others heard about it. We received one and two week's salary contributions from most. A particular registered nurse involved in new patient admittances gave us an entire month's salary. It almost sounds ridiculous that I should continually have to refer to financial difficulties, but that is the way it has been since the inception of the Clinic. Therefore, it is important that the public know what doctors face who want to serve as do those at the Clinic.

With the new year of 1964, we still faced financial problems. One time after a morning emergency meeting, I decided to call Mr. Clement Stone hoping to arrange a meeting in Chicago. I had to tell him about our financial dilemma. When I offered to visit, he wondered why I should travel to Chicago. His reply was, *"Why spend this money to come here when you haven't got it? I am sitting in a very comfortable chair. I'll listen to you as long as you want to talk"* Talk I did. When I finished, he replied, *"How much do you need to meet your payroll at the end of the week and the next one after that?"* I told him I needed $5,000. *"I'll mail it out to you today."* I then told him of the expected deficit in 1964 of $15,000. He promised to send us the balance of money as we needed it.

Perhaps one might ask whether we received contributions from foundations. We did. We do. However it is always in small amounts. For example, for two years, the Permanent Charity Fund gave us one thousand dollars each year.

Aside from foundations, we did not receive profitable help from union welfare funds. We found that unions, such as the Garment Workers and Teamsters, conducted their own clinics. Others purchased their services in some of our largest teaching hospitals. We also invited the representative of the Whiting Milk Company Employees' Union to visit us. When he learned about our medical services he told me that they contract where there is hospitalization.

Yet, we do receive contributions and other support from many unions, the most constant being those with moderate-income laborers, who receive the most benefit and health care through our unique care.

In addition to what I have told above, I must relate about one of the contributions that meant a great deal to us — that from a committee of students organized at Wellesley College for community service allocations. For many years, Wellesley students made an annual contribution of hundreds of dollars, which we valued for their awareness of social responsibility. One memory that I especially treasure is that of an evening about fifteen years ago when, on being invited to speak to the Wellesley student body, I found a waiting audience of young women wanting enlightenment about helping others. Every seat in the hall was taken. Those without seats lay on the floor to listen to our story.

I am often asked, *"How could fine work of this kind, which is such a necessary contribution to health service, not receive sufficient funds to meet its expenses?"* The only answer is that benevolent individuals understood and helped, while others did not. For example, I am thankful that there were those who made large sum contributions to emphasize their faith in our sincerity and purpose. There are people such as Mrs. White, our patient; Mr. Crowell; the Good Neighbor Fund of the General Electric Company; His Eminence Cardinal Richard E. Cushing; Laura Stackpole; and Mr. Clement Stone — it was through his contribution of more than fifty thousand dollars one year which made it possible to keep our doors open to admit our millionth patient.

The most noted fundraising institutions in the country, after visiting and studying the Clinic, told us that we should have no difficulty in raising one quarter of a million dollars. However, we have never been able to pay the fees to hire those large fundraising organizations. For this reason, we continued using the funds we had and could raise in order to operate and to serve.

It may seem like a repetition, but the following is important to note. With the approach of the year 1964, enlightened Americans perceived the inadequacy and downright failure of the medical establishment and those responsible for the planning and for dictating a policy for the creation of health facilities adequate for our entire society. This failure was no longer acceptable to the average American. We pride ourselves on the good life, yet we set such a bad example in health care. European, British, Canadian, and other governments were aware of this need on the part of their citizens — they put in place national health care, while we lag. Even before 1964, recognizing that health care is a national emergency, then President John F. Kennedy thought that surely Congress and the country would go along with his realization, countering the attitude of the medical establishment and the stubbornness of the Congress, which he expected would concur that at least, the 20 million of our citizens over sixty-five should be provided for by law. Of course, he was wrong.

And what was the reason he failed to accomplish what he believed in? It was not that the nation could ill afford it. It seems to me there were insufficient Congressional representatives of the people who would take this message from the President and turn it into a national concern for these millions of citizens. This had to wait for citizens themselves and their cry of indignation. Finally, President Johnson joined his voice to that of the people, which became a chorus, and which finally made Medicare the law of the land. But it is disconcerting to realize that at no time did the established institutions and those who held themselves up as responsible for the health care of all Americans ever exert their efforts on behalf of those who just could not afford the ever-rising costs for which the Establishment was responsible.

At the beginning of 1964, the Clinic trustees reviewed and discussed the effects of Medicare's legislation for the nearly twenty million of our citizens over sixty-five. It appeared to us that our institution and its services for the low/moderate income worker was still an absolute necessity, as the compassionate act of Medicare was not directly beneficial to the health of younger patients. We therefore concluded it was our unavoidable obligation to continue with our service.

One happy reward of our type of service occurred when we received a letter from a youngster treated in the Allergy Department, where the parents were patients too. This youngster got other children in his community to give a show for two cents admission. They then sent a money order for two dollars fifty-eight cents expressing the hope that we *"would put the money to good use to help others."* The writing was in a child's hand.

We were also grateful to be remembered in the legacies of onetime patients for two hundred, four hundred, even a thousand dollars — the largest being a gift from a past patient for twelve thousand. But our largest gifts had to come, as a rule, from wealthier contributors. This indicates that such people must have been informed, in detail, about the services of Healing After Dark. Word-of-mouth and patients' testimonies could not do the whole job. It called for forceful salesmanship, and I really became a good salesman — I've often wondered to what extent the ten-year-old salesman's apprenticeship I had in Romania, at the newspaper corner, and selling the *Standard Dictionary of Facts* served me as basic training to make me as versatile an entrepreneur as I had to become.

CHAPTER ELEVEN: AT THE WHITE HOUSE

In addition to disappointments and struggles, there were honors and encouragements. I have already told of several leaders who honored us; others include James Michael Curley who gave me a key to the City, Governor and Senator Leverett Saltonstall, Governor Christian A. Herter, Mayor John Hynes, our present mayor John Collins, President Dwight D. Eisenhower, President John F. Kennedy, and President Lyndon B. Johnson, who honored me by invitation to become a panel participant at the White House Health Conference in 1965.

In that year, the American Medical Association acknowledged the weak national medical picture. There was a shortage of medical manpower. The Association recognized the need for more medical schools. The new plan called for the establishment of a State medical school. One can imagine the effect on the health care of our citizens, if we failed to address the growing shortage of medical personnel. Regardless of who is responsible for how the shortage came about, the country still lacks at least ten thousand doctors. We are forced to import nearly 10,000 foreign doctors to help fill the need. Yet, this emergency should have been of no surprise to anyone, because it has been inevitable — a logical result of the existing design of public medical care that is blind to the growth of a population in need of health assistance.

Fortunately, President Johnson raised more public awareness for the Medicare Program, for which he has successfully fought. He also called for The White House Conference on Health. I was one of those invited to speak. The invitation came, of course, from the White House, engraved with the Presidential seal and: *"The President of the United States requests the honor of your presence at the White House Conference on Health..."*

Morris A. Cohen, M.D.

The President of the United States

requests the honor of your presence

at the

White House Conference

on Health

at nine o'clock on the mornings of

Wednesday, November third

and Thursday, November fourth

nineteen hundred and sixty five

City of Washington

in the District of Columbia

R.S.V.P.

Regency Ballroom
Shoreham Hotel

The White House Invitation

The entire experience was exceptional, and professionally rewarding. Yet, it wasn't until preparing to leave Washington that I reflected upon the extreme irony of my situation. The paradox was this: to the administrators, as well as to the practitioners, with whom I had met and talked — eight hundred representatives from all over the country — "healing after dark," a clinic established for evening hours, seemed an absolutely novel concept. They were ignorant of our forty years of demonstrated usefulness and of the idea itself. To them, the Clinic that I cultivated all those long years ago was still unexplored ground. Most are still vaguely speculating about such practice as seen in the literature and in discussion groups. The word of our work had not spread beyond the area where patients benefited from it. Acknowledgment of our care for patients during evenings certainly had not been spread by the medical profession.

Now, to my astonishment, I found that there was a national outcry for just such a service. I could not help but recall the visit of Mr. Myles in my office during which he emphasized the importance of our joining the United Community Services, giving as his reason that we were the only health care evening clinic and were not duplicating any other such service in the community. It pleased me simply to know that ultimately, we might be able to make a very great contribution to the welfare of all our citizens, no matter how tardy the publication of its benefits. Our preaching about how we were meeting this challenge — the lack of evening health facilities — was just one immediate way our Clinic might be turned into a national example.

The recommendations I made appeared in the *Congressional Record* of the Committee on Aging, dated January 10 and 20, 1966. During the question period following my comments, one prominent doctor asked me, *"How do you expect the doctors after a day's work to perform efficiently during the evening hours?"* First, I asked him if he was aware of the present necessity of "moonlighting" after regular working hours today in our country, the millions who take second jobs or put in extra time to make both ends meet. For example, a nurse from one of our large hospitals does so by serving two evenings a week at the Clinic to enable her to afford an automobile. I also told him that my reply would provide an example and a question to him, as follows:

"Doctor, we have on our staff one of the busiest orthopedic surgeons in our area. He is on the staff of two teaching hospitals, teaches at a medical school and serves on our staff. One night last winter, a woman fell and was brought into the Clinic. An x-ray wet plate showed a fracture of the radius. It was 9:30 when we looked at the plate. The orthopedic surgeon of whom I speak was still engaged in seeing patients in our Orthopedic Department. I went to him with the x-ray, and believe me, he did look very tired. He undoubtedly had begun operating that morning before eight o'clock. I said, 'Bob, this woman just fell down,' and I presented the plate to him and commented, 'Bob, you look terribly tired.

We could put her in a cab and send her to the emergency ward at Boston City Hospital.' He answered, 'No. I'll be through in a few minutes. I have only one more patient waiting.' Ordering the nurse to prepare a plaster bandage and so forth, he put a cast on the woman's arm. It was 10: 35 p.m. when he finished. Now, my question to you, Doctor, is: 'Do you think that this doctor − from about a quarter to 10 to about 25 minutes to 11 − performed an efficient job for this patient?'"

The positive reactions to my expressions of the philosophy

and practice of Healing After Dark on the various panels of the White House Conference can speak for themselves in one or two more examples.

At dinner in the White House, a retired general, Floyd L. Wergeland, M.D., moved a bit closer to me, took me by the arm, saying:

"Doctor, I am very happy to shake your hand. You have made a great contribution in your preaching of the Evening Clinic overtime hours. Soon after the war, Dr. Cohen, I was in charge of the Walter Reed Hospital. Many of our soldiers failed to come into the clinic for medical needs during the clinic hours. On investigating we found that one had a relative visiting from home; another had an offer to be taken by someone for entertainment, thinking that served very well toward rehabilitation, believing this was more important than coming in to receive clinic treatment. So we started evening clinic service. And we never had one soldier who failed to attend thereafter at the appointed time to receive the care prescribed. So you see, you are making a very, very practical and useful suggestion, and I do hope they realize the value of your recommendation as a solution for the lack of facilities and medical manpower, as well as the assurance that there must be medical care for those who require it."

Another gratifying encounter at the White House was an opportunity to speak with Dr. Comanduras who worked with Dr. Dooley in Laos. After introducing himself, he told me he was enthralled with my recommendations and my concept of Healing After Dark. He said that he was now in charge of the Washington Clinic and expressed the fact that African Americans were among Washington's greatest numbers of people below the moderate wage income level. He then asked if he could have lunch with me at which time he could continue to discuss the organization and clinical administration of our institution. Dr. Comanduras wanted to discuss in greater detail what he heard from me and decided at that time to suggest that such services be made available to those who attend the Washington Clinic.

On my return to Boston, I received many letters from doctors practicing in different sections of the country. Some came to visit with us to inspect our facilities with the idea of starting their own such programs. One doctor who came to see me in Boston was Director of the Health Service Clinics at the Sydney Hillman Health Center in New York. He arrived accompanied by Sadie H. Zaidens, M.D., who was in charge of the Psychiatric Department of that Clinic. She wrote after her visit, *"I wish to thank you for the constructive tour you gave us of your medical center and its psychiatric division in particular. It was very enlightening and I am sure that we shall be able to make use of it in our plans for the Sydney Hillman Health Center. I am planning to do additional work in community psychiatry so that I shall make further use of your experiences in this field."*

It is of interest to read the appraisal of this Conference sent to me by a public-relations person who was present at the session at which I was a speaker. These represent his objective reactions:

A note of caution in expanding government involvement, and a plea for a breathing spell after the unprecedented output of health measures put through the 98th Congress, was sounded by Doctor James Z. Appel, the AMA's new and articulate President.

However, it was Dr. Alonzo S. Yerby, New York City's Hospital Commissioner who seemed most successful in defining the spirit of the Conference. Dr. Yerby made an eloquent appeal for grading medical services to the poor through all means. He charged that "basic medical facilities for America's poor are still... crowded, uncomfortable, and lacking in concern for human dignity; programs are piecemeal, poorly supervised and uncoordinated." He asserted that the poor must no longer be made to "barter their dignity for their health," and described the insurmountable problems confronting a working-class mother who must care for her family through a fragmented system of hospital outpatient specialty clinics which are open at different hours, on different days... Dr. Leona Baumgartner, a Conference Vice-Chairman and Professor of Preventive Medicine and Public Health, expanded in this vein stating the need to "Re- Humanize" what's wrong in medicine after 20 years of technological emphasis and still being unable to deliver these advances to patients in a more meaningful, direct, and effective manner.

One spokesman injected the reminder that soon delegates would return to the same local problems they had left behind. (He might have had the Boston Evening Clinic in mind.) While the Conference helped us to see more clearly the value of our community health programs, and to understand why they must be ipso facto "unprofitable," it did not solve our problem.

The Conference renewed our commitment for the relevance and necessity of evening care for those of limited means... the White House Conference on Health was constructive. It remains to be seen whether the ideas generated there will fulfill the promise, at long last, to abolish for all time the iniquitous two-class health system in this the wealthiest, most advanced society in the world.

At long last a major breakthrough seems possible in providing qualified medical care to the poor. If this happens, the state and federal governments will be in major roles, providing heretofore unparalleled cooperation with private health institutions.

These seem to us the broad results of the historic White House

Conference on Health, November 3-4, 1965, which brought under one roof the nation's most distinguished, influential and knowledgeable health authorities.

Approximately 850 persons were invited by President Johnson from all parts of the country, including such diverse persons as Dr. John Walk, co-developer of the "pill;" Dr. Peter Comanduras co-founder of Medico with the late Tom Dooley; Senator Lister Hill of Alabama; and the mayor of Unalakleet, Alaska.

An impressive delegation from Boston included deans and faculty members from our medical schools, and administrators of several leading hospitals and clinics, including Dr. Morris A. Cohen, founder and Medical Director of the Boston Evening Clinic.

Since the United States is the acknowledged world leader in health it seems reasonable to assert that the Conference represented the most authoritative thinking in the world in the fields of medicine, dentistry, psychiatry, health education, nursing, public health, social work, and so forth.

The thrust of the speakers and reports seemed to be threefold: 1. That minimal adequate health care and protection should be a "right" of citizenship, regardless of race, religion, or ability to pay; 2. That voluntary medical institutions and private practitioners are not equipped to close this gap alone, in terms of planning and allocation of resources, etc.; 3. That the magnitude of the problems (including air and water pollution, professional training, public education, mental illness and retardation, and family planning), require a closer coordination at all levels between voluntary and governmental agencies and resources.

One cannot grasp the significance of these trends in relation to local and national health needs if the attitude is allowed to persist that the so-called "poor" are a residual fringe of unfortunate, somehow not typical of most Americans. In fact, that part today constitutes between 20-30% of our total population, numbering between 40,000,000 and 60,000,000, depending on the criteria for low income that is adopted.

The majority of poor are white. Although the non-white minorities suffer from the most intense and concentrated and impoverishment of any single group.

It must be noted that even as I recall this discussion and read again these notes, the demographics in our nation continue to change rapidly.

In fact, as of 2010, they have indeed changed dramatically. Those below the poverty level of $22,000 per year are at 39.8% of the population, as of this writing in 2010. And the majority consists of African-Americans and those of Hispanic origin. These figures are from the U.S. Census.

— Richard S. Cohen

But to return to the summary of this important meeting:

According to Michael Harrington (in The Other America), "the people who are in this plight add an enormous physical disadvantage, suffering more from chronic disease and having less possibility for treatment. The citizens of the culture of poverty also suffer from more mental and emotional problems than any group in American society."

This is not news to the Boston Evening Clinic, and judging from the spirited ovation to Dr. Morris A. Cohen's plea for expansion of treatment hours in mental health prevention centers, the profession is becoming more cognizant of these facts.

These became days of affirmation of our mission. The time had come at last when I could say to myself that it had all been worthwhile. I and doctors at the Clinic had created and sustained a beneficial new concept of medicine. My efforts brought the wonderful compensation of the spoken "well done" which, emanating from my colleagues in the medical world, gave me tremendous happiness. Speaking to the people that I did and hearing from them was a special reward.

Added to these acknowledgments, I received a letter from Senator Harrison A. Williams, Jr., Chairman of the Special Committee on Aging in the President's War on Poverty as it affects older Americans. He requested that I write my recommendations for him. Now, having become nationally known and having been heard, I felt it was an outstanding opportunity to speak for the American who retains the independent spirit and remains a rugged individual throughout his/her entire life. Senator Edward M. Kennedy, a member of the Committee, also asked me to do the same because the recommendations would be presented before the members in Washington.

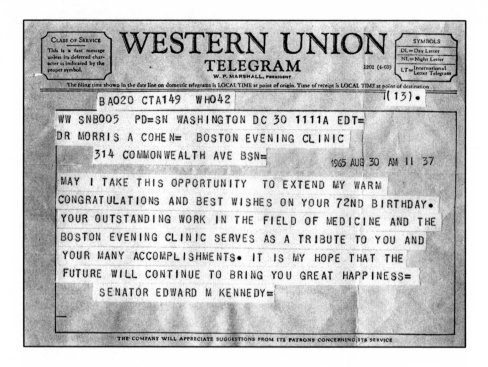

BA020 CTA149 WHO42 ⌐(13)●

WW SNB005 PD=SN WASHINGTON DC 30 1111A EDT=

DR MORRIS A COHEN= BOSTON EVENING CLINIC

314 COMMONWEALTH AVE BSN=

1965 AUG 30 AM 11 37

MAY I TAKE THIS OPPORTUNITY TO EXTEND MY WARM

CONGRATULATIONS AND BEST WISHES ON YOUR 72ND BIRTHDAY●

YOUR OUTSTANDING WORK IN THE FIELD OF MEDICINE AND THE

BOSTON EVENING CLINIC SERVES AS A TRIBUTE TO YOU AND

YOUR MANY ACCOMPLISHMENTS● IT IS MY HOPE THAT THE

FUTURE WILL CONTINUE TO BRING YOU GREAT HAPPINESS=

SENATOR EDWARD M KENNEDY=

Senator Edward Kennedy's congratulatory telegram
to Morris A. Cohen on his 72nd birthday

In the opening statement of my report, I stressed that *"all medical institutions with outpatient facilities" should know the "importance of opening their doors in the evenings, after working hours, so that these people, who are tied by poverty may receive health care at a convenient time." Doing this "means prevention of chronic illness, serious sickness, and prevention of hospitalization and disability."*

My main statement contained these words:

We have since the beginning of our Republic, preached 'rugged individualism,' and these people – these Americans who try so hard under difficult circumstances – should have the opportunity to remain 'rugged individuals' rather than 'ragged individuals.' This is one of our main concerns. We must face up to our national interest and welfare that when over one-third of our working population has an income of less than $3,000 per year and so many of our working population have take-home pay of less than $75 per week, for these people, health is their only asset. Take this away from them and they become your responsibility and mine, and that does become costly and does upset our economic balance and thinking.

The Record continues with two suggestions I made to the White House Conference: that all such institutions throughout the entire country accept the fact that most all of those attending spoke of the lack of medical and paramedical personnel. I brought up the fact that we had lists of medical and paramedical personnel who – through compulsive, economic situations – seek what we call 'moonlighting' work in the evening. I stated that medical facilities should be open not only in the evening, but 24 hours a day, for it is only these institutions that can give care at convenient cost.

The other panel I sat in on was psychiatry. I stated:

We here in this great city of Boston have the only evening ambulatory psychiatric center, which is supported by the State as a community mental health center. One evening we had 90 poor people in this department. Most of them were not psychotic. They have jobs because their therapy keeps them at work and occupied.

They receive meager salaries on these jobs. Thus, they must have psychiatric care in the evenings to continue working.

I want to know – and I am sure you do too – why there are not more of these evening centers to care for these people with mental problems. These are low and moderate wage earners who are not psychotic but have anxieties; they need rest, are confused, and worried and just need kindness and compassion that can mostly be given by trained paramedical personnel, such as psychologists, psychiatric social service workers, psychiatric trained lay people, and the clergy.

Yes, my dear Senator, I am very much interested in your thoughts toward the help of our citizens, particularly those who without help could not be tied to our Great Society of Americans and America. We need them all, for it is they who give up their sons and daughters when danger threatens, and, of course, themselves.

We must think that health is a very, very great factor in our social structure, in our defense, and that it is the very life of our country.

According to the statistics for 1966, outpatient attendance throughout the country was falling as low as fifty percent. It stood to reason that daytime clinics could possibly be neglecting some kind of help which was needed. We stepped up our requests for support so that we could continue to fill that gap; but disappointments, even outrages, still resulted.

To be explicit, let me give you the superficial reaction of a possible large-scale contributor (an industrial leader, who logically should be a civic-minded person) when I asked him to contribute: *"There is just not enough glamour to your institution."* Other leaders have made comments in the same vein. Perhaps there is no answer that allows one to reach the mentality that cannot see the "glamour" of caring for those marginally subsisting. Yet there is something of a miracle for those who visit our Clinic, for they sense immediately when seeing it in operation that it is the stuff of high thrill as compared with the superficial glitter of glamour medicine. Anyone coming to the Clinic can see that paradox.

CHAPTER TWELVE: LAST REFLECTIONS

I have brought the reader through 1966, and the beginning of the present year, 1967. One of my purposes now is to create public awareness and confidence in the public's ability to work at attaining improvements in medical services, as well as to demand the cooperation of fellow citizens in obtaining these improvements, whenever they are not provided by existing agencies.

With the change of civic attitude mostly forced by the informed citizenry under the leadership of our President, we can hopefully look forward to that day in the future, 10 years or more, when we shall have sufficient medical personnel and ancillary services to make possible adequate medical care for all citizens. Hospitals, through federal grants, are improving and enlarging their facilities. New medical schools will open. Many colleges are beginning to include schools for nursing and ancillary technicians.

For the purpose of the new Federal Law P. I. 89-751, referring to the Allied Health Professions Training Act, there will be federal grants to increase the opportunities for the training of medical technologists and allied personnel. Funds will strengthen and improve the existing student loan programs for medicine, dentistry, podiatry, optometry, and nursing students. To accomplish these purposes, the law also matches grants for construction. There are *"improvement grants to help develop new or improved curricula for training. There are loans to schools for the establishment of student loan programs. In addition, the Nurses' Training Act is amended to provide for the establishment of nursing education opportunity grants to assist qualified high school graduates to obtain nursing education."* The institutions representing national medicine, hospitalizations, and other institutions for the sick and the ailing, including the mentally ill, now have the greatest challenge of their existence. They have the opportunity to lend their efforts and abilities in a deserving service to our country and its citizens. They must assist the creative growth of the nation to assure that no American citizen will ever lack adequate health care and thereby keep people sound and productive contributors to their society and country.

In fact, the need is still growing. As of 2010, 40,000 family physicians will be needed by 2020. The figures are from USA Today, by Janice Lloyd. As for foreign trained doctors there are 185,000 such graduates at the present time. The figures are from USA Today, by Greg Suskind.

— Richard S. Cohen

We need to restore our nation to its rightful place as foremost provider to its citizenry of justice and protection in the world, and we must do it by example, by seeing to it that our own citizens can access healing regardless of their financial means.

In 1953, Dr. James Howard Means wrote a book, *Doctors, People and Government.* Associated with the Massachusetts General Hospital, Means wrote, *"All people have a right to medical service, even if they cannot afford to pay... It is among the public duties of the medical profession to seek ways to improve the conditions"* of people.

What astounds me is that just as I have had problems in the past with the Massachusetts Medical Society, Dr. Means described in 1937 how the *Journal of the American Medical*

Association wanted to "impugn [his] motives" and those of thirteen other doctors who presented a twelve-point proposal for the improvement of medical care for Americans. Well, I was, after all, not alone.

Patients appreciated the improvements that the Clinic brought and have often shown their gratitude for kindness. There is this story about a painting. One woman, along in years, a widow with four children to support, made her living scrubbing floors and stairs in office buildings. She had rheumatoid arthritis that we treated for a period of nearly four years. She insisted on paying, and with very great pride kept telling me repeatedly that she was sending one of her sons through college. To her, the cost of working with such pain was her ultimate accomplishment, and helping her son to achieve his goals was compensation enough for her disability. Working throughout the Boston area, she continued coming evenings once a week for gold-therapy injections and other medication. She insisted on paying because she believed if she paid what she could, she was making her own way. She gave us one dollar each visit.

Certainly, this mother must have many times expressed to her son, who painted as a hobby, her gratitude that the Clinic made it possible for her to work, and because of that she was able to continue sending him through college. Or, it may have been that her son, concerned about his mother's circumstances, seeing her every day often in pain, felt the same gratitude as his mother did. After his graduation, with his mother experiencing a respite from pain, the son walked into the Clinic one evening looking for me. He came to express his thanks for his mother's care, realizing that the Clinic was instrumental in his getting a college education. When he came into my office, he was carrying under his arm a framed painting that he had done for me. Ever since that time the painting has hung in my office. It represents a Western scene, a log cabin with a mother holding a child in her arms, and in the roadway a doctor in a horse and carriage is waving goodbye. The symbolism of the subject is unmistakable. What better way may one express gratitude? I see this as just one experience equivalent to the kind of practice I had made up my mind in which to engage. Moreover, that painting perpetually reinforces my efforts.

In addition to patient gratitude and their spreading the word about us, after years of preaching, the public had finally become aware of the necessity of preventive measures, so that we no longer needed to send out sound trucks to attract the public to free care. When even Congressional representatives awakened to this profound public need for prevention, that the medical establishment tried to stop medical intervention is incredible. President Johnson said, *"Our national resources for health have grown but our national aspirations have grown faster. Today we expect what yesterday we could not have envisioned: adequate medical care for every citizen."* Can anyone still wonder why Congress still resists the assurance by law of at least adequate medical care? Do you wonder why some of us in medicine, professionally oriented to a comprehensive view of conditions, looked with favor — despite dissent from some of our medical colleagues — on the overdue legal establishment of Medicare for those sixty-five or over? These are the people who throughout a lifetime of labor contributed their health and strength to help shape and maintain the growing economy and enabled our country to resist all anti-democratic challenges to our way of life. Yet, the AMA stated at that time that no one should interfere with private for-profit medical practice (!) and therefore waged a bitter campaign against Medicare and Medicaid.

It pleases me that since that legislation there has been a more widespread public awareness of the inadequate care and facilities available to those who are inaccurately described as "poor." I am unwilling to call a citizen "poor" when all his/her efforts are focused, under affliction, to avoid becoming a pauper. I may be preaching, but in a democracy only an enlightened and informed citizenry can speak for itself, and it is my hope that the people, through awakened knowledge, will make a cry for health care that all individuals in this nation deserve.

Illustrating my belief that an informed American can speak for himself/herself is an editorial of August 14, 1967. It was in one of the largest circulating Boston newspapers. The editorial was about a moderate income wage earner who picketed the building of the Department of Public Welfare. The editorial stated:

The picket who appeared at City Hall a few days ago with his two small children and a sign demanding tax relief, or, as his sign put it, 'more help for Middle Class Working Man,' has a good case but he picked the wrong villain. His complaint was directed at Welfare Department clients. He noted that his own take-home pay is roughly the equivalent of $155 that is given every two weeks to a welfare mother of five, and he suggested that he is as entitled as she to properly feed and educate his children. Of course he is. But the fact is, that this affluent society has handed both him and the welfare dependent the short end of the stick. The incomes of both are so little above the accepted utter poverty level that neither has a quarrel with the other... an Internal Revenue Service computer discloses that, in his take-home pay and with three dependents besides himself, he is paying $290 per year in income taxes, if he takes the standard deductions. Under the President's proposed 10% war surtax he would pay $319, slightly more than 6 dollars per week. This does not include state income, sales and other taxes.

He may well ask where he is expected to get the money.

The editorial further continued speaking of the low and moderate wage earners who are trying under dire circumstances not to accept welfare for themselves and those dependent upon them in order to make both ends meet. They are only seeking their fair share.

Finally, however, the less fortunate people are learning to speak for themselves or are finding a voice which can be heard in the White House and in Congress. I refer not only to forty million recipients of welfare but also of the citizens on the job every day. The editorial cited above also stated that a third of our workforce is in the same circumstances as the man to which the column referred.

These people about whom I write have been ignored entirely too often by those who administer services to them. For example in the book *Health Care Is A Community Affair*, by Marion B. Folsom, one finds an unpleasantly revealing statement of insensitivity. In a comment on basic findings of a National Commission on Community Health Services, he points to millions who cannot afford care and states that should the Government have to pay for these people, there is a large tax loss.

Obviously, I disagree. A healthy society where all are given health care contributes to the national economy, making the tax argument invalid. There are also a number of informed leaders of government, regardless of political party, who would disagree and who saw value in the Clinic services. For example, Governor John A. Volpe reappointed me Trustee of the Massachusetts Mental Health Center.

Governor Foster Furcolo appointed me to serve for seven

more years. We now have in Massachusetts, by creation of law, paid community mental health centers. The State is divided into two hundred thirty-seven regions, thus assuring mental health care for those of low and moderate wages. At the head of the program is *preventive* mental health care, bearing out my precept that if these millions of our citizens could receive preventive care at convenient times, and for reasonable fees, they would more probably avail themselves of timely care and prevent chronic, possibly irreversible mental incapacity, or even other diseases and hospitalization.

To bring this picture up to date, I refer the reader's attention to the advent of deinstitutionalization – not that there weren't many reasons for it – but also the inadequacy of the alternative care model which was proposed but never fully enacted, the outpatient clinic system – the results with which society now contends: crime and homelessness. Also now, in 2009 and 2010 and in spite of the statistics having worsened from the ones cited earlier by Morris – Congress, including the House and the Senate, argued whether the people "deserve" government sponsored health care, mindless that we are so badly remiss in comparison to all other westernized countries. This argument was forwarded especially by the Republican Party, the insurance companies, and corporate America, all of whom used the asinine and misleading argument that it would be "socialistic" – in spite of the fact that Congress itself and the elderly already enjoy such care. Another aspect of this sad picture is that the "sudden, fearsome medical bills" do occur with regularity among these low-income groups, with devastating results, especially when the economy cannot support them either; families with children end up in shelters, dependant upon charity. Yet a large segment of the population continues to blindly "believe" that these are undeserving people who accept charity out of laziness. Another ignorant, invalid argument is against taxation, which too many of our elected officials support merely out of fear of losing the support of their constituencies. Thus many Americans — who are taxed less than almost all other progressive nations — continue to resent asking those who can afford it to help service those who cannot. Most westernized countries have found a way to provide health care for all without placing any inordinate burden on their nations' economies, and in fact they have found that a healthier citizenry contributes to that economy to a greater extent. Before the Health Care bill was enacted under President Obama, Massachusetts already had a similar health plan, which much of the country looked at as a model. Amazingly, it has taken until the 21st century for this to occur, long after Dr. Cohen wrote the words regarding the Mental Health Program.

— Richard S. Cohen

There is a question I was often asked by leading citizens: "How do you expect to continue under such stress and lack of funds?" My answer always is, "We will continue until such time as others begin to do what we have done — which I see as perhaps the most necessary kind of health care to provide for the moderate/low wage earner, whose one million admittances resoundingly validate this work." I shall continue to practice medicine in this way until many others have heard that my exertions have not only been worthwhile but that those others in the medical profession should open their facilities evenings and after working hours. As stated in the Congressional Record, in answer to a question from a famous industrial leader (who also served as a Trustee of a leading medical institution in our community), I asked: "Why is *your* institution — having facilities and equipment costing nearly three hundred million dollars — *not* being opened for service in the evening?"

There is one other issue I need to address. It has never been the Clinic's intention to serve those in the higher income groups. We have, however, served a handful of higher-income persons when it was absolutely necessary to offer them comprehensive care or diagnostic services, particularly in our cancer detection department, or in the psychiatric department where a long, intensive two-year care was necessary; but these were exceptions and very few in number.

Recently, a first-time visitor who had come to observe the Clinic's operations set down his reactions in a number of notes. The following uncorrected account should help visualize a Clinic evening:

Outside, individuals, couples, small groups come and go; cabs parked legally or otherwise, picking up and dispensing others. A quiet, purposeful bustle inside, for a shock is the number and variety of people who were seated, receiving answers at one or another desk, coming and going on the stairs up, and to the diagnostic services below. Later, on a quickie tour, this shock is deepened by discovery that there are high off a dozen other collection points where large numbers of other people are also waiting and conferring at the ante-rooms to various of the departmental clinics (Cancer Detection, Allergy, Dentistry, X-ray, etc.).

Impressions of people-to-people interaction:

Two older women in house dresses, one small, the other large and extremely wan-complected, she sits heavily next to a stranger. Her friend cheerfully shuffles two paper cups of water from the nearby cooler. To the receptionist she tells she is entering a hospital following morning. ("Gee this is good water.")

A young couple comes by to get the results of chest plates made the previous week. People enter, stopped briefly at the desk, scribble a few words and disappear, obvious familiarity of their surroundings in one direction or another. It is quite obvious this is their clinic. New patients are quickly made to feel a part of it, and that it is treated with loving respect. It is obvious that many people are worried, that they are awaiting test results of examinations and are fearful of the results; but it is equally clear that everyone knows this and is a little bit more considerate of one another than might otherwise be the case; and that despite the serious reason for being at the clinic that these people are purposeful, happy, and above all jealously grateful of the Clinic's existence.

The Boston Evening Clinic is not a good Clinic; it is a great one. That is not something one can judge just by looking (although Boston Evening Clinic has all the 'papers' required for top-flight accreditation). It is in the much abused words 'dedicated people'. We have been deafened by the meaning of such words, and are reminded forcibly over what is their literal meaning here at the BEC. Why 'dedicated', in any sense beyond that of any professional calling? It clearly stems from the example of one man, the founder and Medical Director, Dr. Morris A. Cohen, who at 72, is busier than a straw boss in pickin' time with a kind word for a patient, a direction for a doctor, a few of his own examinations, and is in constant motion up and down the six flights of marble stairs. People know that he renounced a career that promised worldly comforts to start the clinic in 1927. They know he likes each and every patient who comes, they know he is putting in his 'second day' at the Clinic.

I am often asked why I still work into the late hours of 9 or 10 p.m. It is because of the patients, obviously, and because of those mentioned above and their contributions. These are reason enough. When asked, "How do you continue to run up and down the stairs after so many hours?" My answer is always, "I'm having a good time doing it. This is the work I love." And this no doubt helps keep my energies at a high level.

With my long working days, the reader may wonder when I rest. Well, the exceptional place that gives me renewal among all the problems is my home, always filled with beauty and the music my wife loves, and a wife who knows I must eat at irregular hours and then relax. To stop me from thinking about Clinic problems during dinner, she reads to me from what she knows will interest me. There is also always a list of periodicals, with marked pages to read, spread out near my bedside, especially on the weekends when there is more time. We live simply, never requiring much, and there were many times we did not have that much. However my wife has a wonderful knack and love of making our home seem lavish in its warmth. She enjoys making her own dresses, sews beautifully. There are times when I have to go to speak at an affair, and she wears an evening gown she made that I am always proud of. The public should also see our yard and the garden she has created. People stop to admire it when walking by. I am fortunate because she has given me the kind of home and life that has strengthened me for the work that I will continue as long as possible.

My philosophy was borne out at the very inception of the Clinic by the influence of a good physician, an elderly man who joined with us, feeling that we had started a new kind of practice for a large and neglected group of our fellow men and women. Pleased that we shared his own spirit of giving, he stated his philosophy as a legacy from a man with years of practice and wisdom. He told me, "You put your arms around your patients, and you will cure most of them." This is a dynamic truth. What the doctor was expressing was the compassion that the medical profession should have for humanity. In truth, if a patient is humiliated, even medical science will find it difficult to affect a cure. It is also what Justice Adlow said in his speech to the West Enders when he talked of family love and care as a preventive in the past for psychiatric problems.

I have read a reference to the outstanding humanitarian, Dr. Albert Schweitzer, in whose philosophy the aim of serving humankind is paramount. He said, *"The destiny of man is to become more and more human."* We see this also stated in other terms by a nun: *"The greatest sin of man is the practice of non-concern for his neighbor."* Concern for our neighbors is the concept upon which the Clinic was founded. If staff members ignored this belief, as it was by a few, I asked them to discontinue their service at the Clinic.

It is a pleasure now to speak of happy days, now that the medical approval agencies, and other institutions such as the welfare and social service agencies, have accepted the Clinic. This group also includes civic-minded citizens working for the betterment of the country. Now, we were at last debt-free for the first time and progressing in our work.

As I have said, the Conference and visitors to the Clinic, as well as the expressions of people from within and outside the country was a reward beyond anything I could have imagined. Moreover, I have tried to convey to the reader the gift of appreciation of the good things of life, the values of life, and the gift of giving.

If this is preaching, what better sermon can I offer but my story and myself? For that has been the reason for my message. To have good health at the age of seventy-three enables one to continue to do what he loves and wills himself to do. And good health is tremendously dependent upon contentment. A contented life gives one stability, strength, and health, for the days and years are never then unnecessarily disturbed by emotional conflict. Very few of us get the opportunity in life to do what we love as a lifetime occupation. I have been one of those fortunate.

I have also been very fortunate in my origins. Although there were no doctors to lead the way for me, I did have hard working, honest, loving parents. They were all I needed as examples. As proof let me again present my mother. Her name was Epta, i.e. *the happy personality.* Always smiling, always singing, and calm, her photograph still smiles at me from a bookcase shelf. She sang the songs of love that she remembered from childhood. They were Romanian songs, gay and spirited. I sang one of these songs only very recently at the wedding of my grandson, Martin, who just reached his second year at George Washington University Medical School. It was an appropriate moment for hearing these Romanian words, because the bride Susan's father had recently learned the Romanian language and will soon be on his way as First Secretary, Economics Advisor of the American Embassy in Bucharest. My words were a surprise to him. And I was singing with the feeling that my mother was standing beside me, singing the song she taught me. She was a good person. In the latter years of her life, there were always at least a dozen boxes marked with the names of each of her many charities in the various rooms of her home. She had days when she would collect funds in the community to donate to these various charities.

I remember another wedding of a cousin on a Sunday, five days before the passing of my mother, when she was singing to the gathering a song she had loved and taught me too. What a duet that was! On the Friday following the wedding, a date before a holiday, at about 5:30 a.m., I received a call from my mother that she was very ill. I called a doctor friend to meet me at her home. The previous three days before the holiday she had been walking throughout the community and up many flights of stairs to collect money for her charities. I often remember the many times she dug into my pocket to take money to pay for a charity lunch or dinner she was to attend. I remember her sitting up in bed smiling at me and saying she knew that she was to die. The doctor and I tried awfully hard to prolong her life; but after four hours of trying, she looked at me smilingly and uttered something which sounded to me like *"God be with you,"* and she closed her eyes.

I am reminded of being at another bedside death, that of my father, who was so proud of his doctor son. In his last effort, he sat up, put his hands upon my shoulders, and looking at me, he too tried to say goodbye with the same blessing, *"God be with you."*

Well, I have contented but tragic memories of the passing years, my parents, who gave so much and were so happy in the deeds and missions in which they involved themselves. They passed that happy nature on to me. Moreover, the discipline, love, and reverence practiced and instilled by these parents served me as an example in creating the character of my own children.

I have tried to present myself honestly. Remember, too, that there is a price to pay for all the things one values and wishes to possess or accomplish. The work of the institution to which I have dedicated the entire productive years of my life was my way of giving, and the blessings I *knew* and felt. I have also tried to reawaken the hopeful spirit of living in the United States that is still the land of freedom and opportunity, to tell how good deeds for human beings repay a person no matter how hard the labor. This has been the core belief of my life.

155

EPILOGUE by Richard S. Cohen

On a summer afternoon in 1971, sitting on a sun porch talking politics, war, and family, suddenly Morris Aaron Cohen, husband and father, looked at his wife Chloe, and at my wife Arla and me. "I'm thinking seriously of retiring. They've asked me to. Maybe I should."

Who was "they?" Well, it wasn't a large majority of the Board — but a close relative and perhaps two or three others.

Chloe had heard this talk before and sometimes wished he would just get out of the Clinic altogether and be home in his backyard, admiring her magnificent garden. There were times she despised the Clinic, and early in the marriage she regretted not having more time with Morris. But as time went on, this faded. What bothered her was the pain the Clinic often caused him. In some ways, I suppose one could say she agreed with my mother's assessment. Undeniably, however, the Clinic never took from Chloe's life, as it had from my mother's. Of course there were times I compared the two women. However, for me the Clinic was like a twin.

I never agreed with Chloe when she wanted my father to stop. It annoyed me, perhaps, having grown up with the Clinic. So, during our conversation, I immediately objected. "You can't do that. It would no longer be the Clinic."

Does one man make an institution? Well, not always. But my father and that institution always seemed to me to be inseparable. He and it caused many problems within the family, but that they should be severed seemed an abomination. My father and the Clinic were one and the same.

He looked at Chloe. She hesitated. "Morris, you won't be happy. You won't want to see what happens after you leave."

"Dad," I said, "forget it."

There is no question when you looked at my father that the years of struggle showed. In fact, one day I asked him, "Are you O.K.?" In his usual way, he glanced at me. "Yes." You learned with my father that when he answered that way, there were to be no more questions.

The retirement discussion on the sun porch finally ended with his resolution to stay. Being family, one could not imagine how the Boston Evening Clinic could be what it became without him still sitting as Medical Director. In fact, events proved this true. This was a man with willpower, with a magnificent mind, with inborn charm, and with strong discipline — with which he controlled not only himself but also, as I found out quite young, his children, to a point.

At this time, I was a member of the Board of Trustees along with my brother, George M. Cohen (we kidded him about his name, for he did write lilting, romantic songs, though he never tried to publish them for some reason). My father's brother Bill was also a member. He came on for his business skills, so we were told; at the age of fifty he had retired a wealthy man from a senior insurance executive position.

And then retirement became a subject once more. This time was in 1973, again summer. Arla and I were home from Illinois where I was Chairman of the English and Speech Department at Illinois Benedictine University in Lisle. On one particular day, I walked into my father's office. He sat at his desk preparing for the Board meeting we were soon to attend.

He looked up, smiled, "Hi."

"Hi." I always looked about the office, the bookcases, the photos of my brothers in their World War II uniforms, the White House Invitation on the wall, along with other photos and framed letters. The desk, immaculate, always held a pipe or two, depending on whether one was in his mouth.

"I'm going down to the meeting and tell them I resign," he announced.

"You can't do that."

"Well, Bill thought I should." Bill was younger than my father, of course, but because of his successful career, the feeling was that his judgment regarding the Clinic was sound for any kind of business.

I sat with my father and insisted he not give up. We talked for a while, he agreed, and we went down.

As in other Boardrooms, there was a long table at which sat the trustees. There was the usual chatter and some meaningful work done. Then the Chair said, "Dr. Cohen has something he wishes to tell the Board."

My father stood up. He had a sense of timing and dramatics as good as any actor, stage or screen. Without hesitation, looking at my uncle, then at the Chairman, he said: "I thought I would offer my resignation today. Well, I will not." He sat.

More memorable was the expression on my uncle's face and on the faces of the few others who had been hoping he would retire. Astonishment. It amused me.

When we left the room, my father appeared rather self-satisfied. "That settles that," was all he said, and we returned to his office.

So what kind of father was Morris Aaron Cohen? Well, he did start something of a medical dynasty. He also had an influence on some of those who followed. His eldest son Manley became a thoracic surgeon. When he practiced in El

Paso, he was one of the only doctors who would operate and see patients at the El Paso City Hospital. Few would ever think of being Chief of Staff. Manley never hesitated. Why? Because the people were poor Hispanics. I also remember once in the surgeons' dressing room at one of the bigger hospitals one of the "well-known" surgeons not only making fun of Hispanics but damning "Niggers." I can never forget my surprise and disgust regarding him and several other white doctors who were much the same.

After the war George worked at the Clinic and began his own optometric practice in Cambridge, then practiced in Gloucester, Massachusetts for about forty years, retired, and died there in 1997. And I, the youngest son, although I made a career in literature and academic administration, did medical research after my WWII army service.

As to the next generation: Manley's son Myles won international recognition in hand surgery, on which he is the author of a text; he serves on the Board of Cedar-Sinai Hospital in Los Angeles, where he was Medical Director, Chief of Surgery and where he has practiced for many years. Alfred's son Martin, a gastroenterologist, practiced in the large Amarillo Diagnostic Clinic, in Texas. His awards include Best Doctors in America, Guide to America's Top Physicians, Top Doctors in Texas, and the Cambridge University, England award: Leading Health Professionals in the World. He has also become known for his excellence in photography, for which he has won prizes and has been exhibited in a number of galleries. And my own son, Mylan, a noted nuclear cardiologist, in 2010 was President of the Association of Nuclear Cardiologists. I once asked Mylan whether my father influenced him. He told me my dad did but more so, my step uncle Aeneas, Chloe's brother who we used to visit, practiced in the small town of Harrisville, Michigan. Mylan was older then and was fascinated, I imagine, not only by Aeneas but by the way he practiced medicine and took care of everyone. I do know Myles and Martin were fascinated by my father's lifetime dedication to his profession and the people he served.

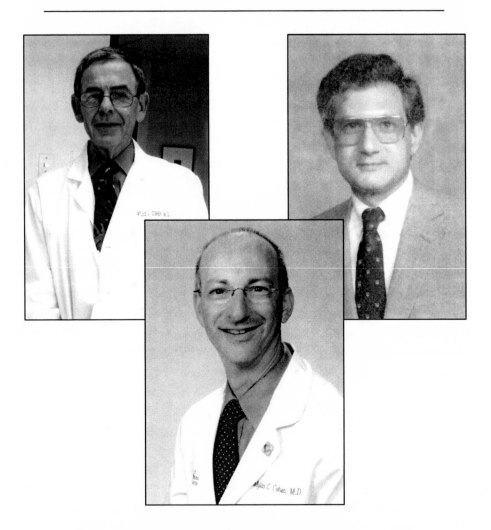

Clockwise from top left: Myles J. Cohen, M.D., A.S.S.H.;
Martin I. Cohen, M.D., A. C. G.;
Mylan C. Cohen, M.D., M.P.H., F.A.C.C.

There's one thing I know for certain: that despite the conflicts he endured in the Clinic and at home, the sacrifices and the penalties, my father always cared deeply for his children, though there were times some of us may have not seen it expressed in the way we might have wished. However, when there were problems, I remember times when he would gather my brothers and consult with them, as though he were at a board meeting.

Is this information necessary in the story of Morris Cohen's life and that of the Clinic? Yes. There are always varying sides of a public individual, as the public sees him, as seen privately. I have inserted my family memories and Clinic stories in the hopes that these serve to fill in the outline of this very extraordinary individual, complex because of his unshakable sense of mission.

The death of my father occurred on February 22, 1974, at age eighty-one, when I lived in Illinois. We had come to Boston by train from Chicago, because my father had cancer, and was in the then Peter Bent Brigham Hospital. My brother George had called to tell me our father was slipping away. At the hospital, we went to his private room, seeing a pallid, gray haired man partially asleep. I leaned over the railing. "Dad." He opened his eyes, looked, then spoke very softly, "What are you doing here?"

"Well, I was on my way to Washington for the school and decided to stop so we could see you." (A lie of course, even though I did take such trips).

"That's good." He watched me through pain-blurred eyes. Softly again, "Why are you going?" I told him it was about a grant. We did that sometimes too. "It was good of you to stop by," and he firmly grasped my hand. It was difficult trying to hide the tears.

After leaving him, I talked to his doctor who told me that the prognosis was bad. At the beginning of this Epilogue, I told how I had asked my father if he was O.K. Well, the lie was there in a hospital bed.

We took the train back to Chicago and then to Naperville where we lived. A couple we knew was taking care of the children. The husband met us at the train and almost immediately told me, "Your brother called and wanted you to call as soon as you came home." The call was an obvious message. When I spoke to George he told me our father died during the night. In fact, I have thought of the irony. I saw him the day before and while we were sleeping on the train that night, my father had died.

The running of the Clinic was picked up by, I understood, my uncle Bill, a nurse, and another woman.

During that summer, I was offered the position of Assistant Vice-President of Academic Affairs at the University of Maine at Presque Isle. Before going there, a meeting was held at the Clinic of the Board of Trustees, and I attended. It is difficult to remember what the agenda actually was. At some point, however, a motion was made. I raised my hand and challenged them: "You cannot do what you are trying here. Haven't you all read the by-laws?" Whatever was going to happen stopped. The members looked at me. "Well, haven't you all ever read them?" No one then on the Board had, apparently. The meeting ended not long after. One of the members came to me and said "I hope you will continue to come to meetings."

Shortly afterwards, I received a call from my brother George asking me to resign from the Board in solidarity with him — he had already done so, in protest of what was happening. My mistake was that I did so. That was not just my error but his also. One of the women, I believe, became Director, and, so far as I know, my uncle continued to be her advisor.

Eventually, at the city's urging that there be centers such as the Boston Evening Clinic throughout the Boston area, the hospitals at last took leadership. Massachusetts General Hospital bought the Boston Evening Clinic. The nurse from the Clinic was given a position by the Massachusetts General in an office titled the Boston Evening Clinic Foundation. To the best of my knowledge, there were deserving funds distributed to good medical organizations or individuals, one of which I have knowledge.

Morris A. Cohen did not really die, however. Obviously, he lives in his children and grandchildren, but more so in those of his profession who followed his example anywhere that compassionate health care was offered regardless of ability to pay. And I might add, in the spirit and determination of the people in 2010, Congress finally managed to pass a Health Care bill, the Affordable Care Act, which begins to extend healing to all.

– Richard S. Cohen

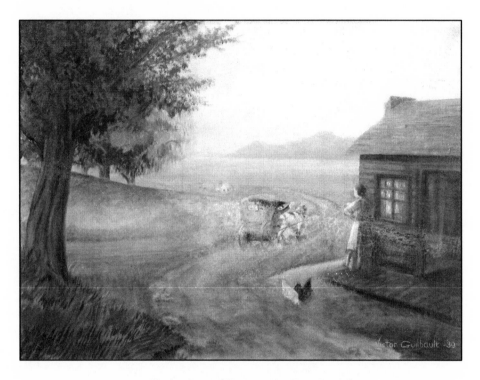

Painting of Doctor in Buggy

Color version of painting may be viewed in e-book edition or at:

www.ccbpublishing.com/rscohen.html

or

www.richardshaincohen.com

INDEX

Danforth, Pitt W., 38, 49, 75
Dean, Ernest, 47, 48
Department of Hygiene, 119
Department of Public Health, 104, 105, 119, 146
Doctor and Buggy Painting, 164
Dooley, Doctor Tom, viii, 132, 135

East Side, New York City, 23
Eisenhower, President Dwight D., 128
El Paso, Texas, 16, 85, 158-159
Elie, Rudolph, 88
Ellsworth, Doctor, 35
Embden Pond (Lake), Maine, 97, 98, 100
England, 84, 125
Ethics and Discipline, Committee on, 36, 43, 45, 56, 57, 59, 60

Fall River, Massachusetts, 17
Faneuil Hall, Boston, 14
Feldman, Doctor Louis, 32
First National Bank of Boston, 73, 118
Fitchburg, Massachusetts, 19
Folsom, Marion B., Health Care Is A Community Affair, 147
Frechette, Doctor. Alfred, 106
Friend Street, Boston, 14
Furcolo, Governor Foster, 58, 111, 112, 147

Gallagher, Doctor (Ph.D.) Eugene, B., 109
Gannon, Mrs., 51, 62
Garment Workers of America, 124
George Washington Medical School, 154
Gloucester, Massachusetts, 83, 159
Golden, Doctor Harry, 33, 43
Good Neighbor Fund, 125
Grages, Harry, 66

Granger, Doctor Frank B., 35
Green and Chardon Streets, Boston, 11
Gridley's in Pie Alley, 8
Grover, Sam, 14

Hamel, Henry E., 67
Harrington, Michael, The Other America, 136
Harrisville, Michigan, 159
Harry and Louise ad, x
Harvard Glee Club, 51
Harvard Medical School, 42, 111
Harvard University, 16
Health Care Reform Bill (Affordable Health Care Act), 149, 163
Health Department, City of Boston, 64
Henderson, Ernest, 74
Hendrix Club, 11
Hereford Street, Boston, 114
Herter, Governor Christian, 128
Higgins, Judge, 11
Hill, Senator Lister, 135
Hollywood, 18
Hood Rubber Company, 65
Hospital Council of Metropolitan Boston, 103, 120
Hudson River, 20
Hynes, Governor John, 128

Illinois Benedictine University, 157
Industrial Medical Association, 97
Influenza Epidemic, 1918, 24

JA Cigar Company, 64
Jassy, Romania, 4, 5
Jessel, George, 17
Jewish Advocate, The, 122
Johnson, President Lyndon B., viii, 1, 3, 44, 106, 126, 128, 135, 145, 146
Jones, William, 47
Jonsson, Mr., 49

Parkman Street, West End, Boston, 27
Permanent Charity Fund, 76, 124
Peter Bent Brigham Hospital, Boston, 59, 161
Philadelphus, Ms., 68
Phinney, Mr., 115, 116
Phoenix Mutual Insurance Company, 114, 119
Podu-lloi, Romania, 3, 4, 5
Pogrom, 5
Police Station 16, Boston, 35
Portland, Maine, x
Post Graduate Institute of the Massachusetts Medical Society, 120
Providence, Rhode Island, 17
Psychiatric Department of the Clinic, 109, 119, 121
Psychiatric Quarterly Supplement, 109
Public Health, Massachusetts Department of, 54, 58, 120
Public Welfare, Massachusetts Department of, 41, 54, 55

Reconstruction Hospital, New York, 35
Redpath, Mrs., 69
Reno, Nevada, 81
Republican Party, 148
Roche, Arthur, 76
Romania, 3, 5, 6, 7, 60, 127
Roosevelt, Anna, 77
Roosevelt, Franklin D., President, 72, 77

Salerno, Italy, 83
Saltonstall, Senator Leverett, 48, 128
Sawyer, Frank, 38, 49
Sawyer's Market, North Anson, Maine, 100
Schweitzer, Doctor Albert, 153

Scollay Square, Boston, 7
Shain, Doctor Joseph, 62, 63
Shain, Jessica (m. Lavine), 79
Simmons College, 79
Smith, Doctor L.C., 45
Snow, Doctor William Benham, 35
Solomon, Doctor Harry C., Commissioner of Mental Health, 58, 119
South Ashburnham, Massachusetts, 17, 18, 19
Southampton, England, 6
Spanish Count, 22, 23
Special Committee on Aging, 137
St. Joseph's Church, Boston, 27
Stackpole, Laura McKinley, 113, 125
Stander, Doctor Alvin, 120
State Budget Director, 119
State Department of Public Health, Massachusetts, 104, 105, 106, 120
Stone, Clement, 123, 125
Stone, Doctor Elizabeth, 47
Stratton, Doctor, 78
Sydney Hillman Health Center, New York, 133

Teamsters Union, 124
"This is Your Life", 107
Thorndike, Doctor Augustus, 33
Time Magazine, 18
Times Square, New York City, 21
Tobin, Governor Maurice, 90
Town Taxi Company, 32
Truman, Harry, President, 90

Unalakleet, Alaska, Mayor of, 135
Union Square, New York, 20
United Community Services, 101, 102, 103, 130
United Fund, 101,102
United States Census, 136
United States Congress, 126, 133, 145, 147, 148

United States Senate, 148
University of Maine at Presque Isle,
    162
USA Today, vi, 143

Veterans' Administration Clinic, 109,
    110
Vienna, Austria, 6
Vigoda, Morris, 69
Volpe, Governor John A., 58, 147

Waldorf Restaurant Chain, 17
Walk, Doctor John, 135
Walker, Doctor Irving, 33
Walter Reed Hospital, 132
War on Poverty, 1, 137
Washington Clinic, 132, 133
Washington, District of Columbia,
    130, 132, 161
Ways and Means Committee,
    Massachusetts, 119
Wellesley College, 124
Wergeland, General Floyd L., 132
West End Old Timers, 11, 153
West End, Boston, 6, 8, 11, 27, 32
Wheeler, Doctor William D., 33, 57
White House Conference on Health,
    viii, 128, 134
White House, 147, 157
White, Mrs., 125
Whiting Milk Company Employees'
    Union, 124
Wilinsky, Doctor Charles, 64
Williams, Jr., Senator Harrison A.,
    137
Women of Means, x
Workman's Compensation, 29, 30
World War I, 18
World War II, 18, 83, 84, 85
Wright, Bishop, 67

Yerby, Doctor Alonzo S., 133, 134

Zaidens, Doctor Sadie H., 133
Zazu Pitts, 17
Zieman, Irving, 91